Mental Health Worldwide

Mental Health Worldwide

Culture, Globalization and Development

Suman Fernando

Faculty of Social Sciences and Humanities, London Metropolitan University, UK

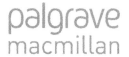

First published 2014 by
PALGRAVE MACMILLAN

Palgrave Macmillan in the UK is an imprint of Macmillan Publishers Limited, registered in England, company number 785998, of Houndmills, Basingstoke, Hampshire RG21 6XS.

Palgrave Macmillan in the US is a division of St Martin's Press LLC, 175 Fifth Avenue, New York, NY 10010.

Palgrave Macmillan is the global academic imprint of the above companies and has companies and representatives throughout the world.

Palgrave® and Macmillan® are registered trademarks in the United States, the United Kingdom, Europe and other countries.

ISBN 978–1–137–32959–2 hardback
ISBN 978–1–137–32958–5 paperback

This book is printed on paper suitable for recycling and made from fully managed and sustained forest sources. Logging, pulping and manufacturing processes are expected to conform to the environmental regulations of the country of origin.

A catalogue record for this book is available from the British Library.

A catalog record for this book is available from the Library of Congress.

*To my family in England and Sri Lanka, in particular
my grandsons Nathan and Alec*

Contents

Tables

Acknowledgements

I am indebted to the works of scholarship in the fields of anthropology, psychiatry, psychology, religion and sociology, especially those works that cut across disciplines. Further, I derived much stimulation for writing this book from discussions with people who have used mental health services and colleagues of various disciplines in the UK, Canada, The Netherlands and Sri Lanka; and from insights I gained while working in Sri Lanka between 2007 and 2011 with valuable support and encouragement from Duncan Pedersen and Laurence Kirmayer of McGill University, Montreal, Canada. Finally, I am grateful to Nicola Jones and the editorial team at Palgrave Macmillan for their support during the process of writing this book; and most of all the patience and support of my wife Frances.

Introduction

This book is about mental health worldwide—across the globe. I decided not to use the term 'global' in the main title for the following reasons: First, the concept of 'globalization' in the field of mental health means different things to different people—a matter discussed in Chapter 1. Second, the term 'global mental health' has been popularized and pushed recently as a new and special subject, causing confusion by linking mental health development to the imposition of global solutions to mental health problems everywhere; doing so by using terms such as 'scaling up' (services) and 'evidence-based practice' that imply an ideology that (western) psychiatry and psychology have all the answers and that there is very little space for sociology, anthropology, religion and philosophy, and no place at all for non-western medical systems, philosophies, religions and healing.

This book presents evidence on why a *global* approach to mental health and the development of mental health services is mistaken and dangerous; moreover, it presents a critical view of what has happened in the past and what could happen in the future if we are not careful. But more importantly, the book presents an alternative approach whereby services are developed *locally*, cognizant of the fact that the meaning of mental health is culturally and socially determined. There are a variety of *perceptions* worldwide about mental health and illness and various *perspectives* worldwide to consider when mental health services are planned or delivered; for example, the culturally diverse meanings of 'mental health', evidence of people who use the services and the social and political context in which development takes place. In other words, there is neither a global meaning of 'mental health' nor a model of service provision that fits all locations, countries and cultural groups. And, in the case of what may be identified as 'illness' of the mind, there are no *global* remedies. If mental health services are to be relevant, fair and sustainable, they must be fashioned in association with *local* communities, taking on board what *local* people want and need. Nobel Laureate Amartya Sen (1999) says that the 'central part of the exercise of development' is to overcome a variety of problems that affect people in both rich and poor countries; and it is important in all development work to give recognition 'to the centrality of individual freedom *and* to the force of social influences on the extent and reach of individual freedom' (1999, pp. xi–xii, emphasis in original).

As in some of my previous books on mental health, I take a historical approach to understanding current global perspectives on mental health. I start with a short chapter (Chapter 1) on culture and globalization before going on (in Chapter 2) to draw a picture in broad outline of the variety of (culturally determined) traditions towards mental health that have emerged in the world in the past and underpin much of mental health thinking today. Then, I work through various stages to finally discuss in Chapter 8 how things stand today, before venturing to suggest (in Chapter 9) changes in mental health services that could improve experiences of people who access services in the rich countries of the Global North and (in Chapter 10) guidelines on how best mental health development in the Global South should be approached so that local people there have better mental health and well-being in the future (see below for discussion of terms such as 'Global North' and 'Global South').

In researching the field that the book covers, I found that most of the English-language literature was about mental health issues in Europe and North America and about people of European heritage and cultural background in Australia and New Zealand. Also, I found hardly anything relevant in the English-language literature that I could access about current mental health work in South America and very little about indigenous practices in places outside Europe that have been settled en masse by Europeans. Although the book undoubtedly suffers from these limitations, in my view, there is sufficient material from across the world to draw on to make some sense of a complex field and come to definite conclusions.

Some points about language

I try to keep the language in this book as 'ordinary' as possible. I avoid using technical words that may be understandable only to particular professional groups, abstruse arguments and complicated sentences. Also, I try not to get bogged down in discussions of the nitty-gritty of complex issues but, instead, focus on addressing the large picture (for example, the 'politics' of mental health) and practicalities (for example, how mental health services may affect the lives of ordinary people) so that some conclusions can be drawn that apply now. But there are some problems of language that do not go away.

The terminology for describing groups of countries worldwide has changed over the years. William Easterly (2006), former economist at the World Bank and Professor of Economics at New York University, finds that the idea of 'The White Man's Burden', coming from a poem written in 1899 by Rudyard Kipling, underpinned 'a theme throughout history [since the European Enlightenment] of the West and the Rest' (p. 19). Civilization was imagined as being brought by the former to the latter. After the Second World War (WWII),

> self-rule [in former colonies] and decolonization became universal principles. The West exchanged the old racist coinage for a new currency. 'Uncivilized' became 'underdeveloped'. 'Savage peoples' became the 'third world'. There was a genuine change of heart away from racism and toward respect for equality, but a paternalistic and coercive strain survived. (pp. 20–21)

I am not so sure about the change of heart going very deep, but certainly today, ex-colonial nations profess adherence to human rights and the rule of law with respect for national sovereignty, rather than domination by force of arms. Whether they keep very closely to these professed standards is another matter.

The various terms used in this book referring to groups of countries reflect historic, political and economic contexts in the world since the end of WWII. 'Third World' (Tomlinson, 2003) was applied to those countries that refused to be aligned to either of the two power blocs (communist and western) during the Cold War that followed the end of WWII. As ex-colonial countries began to look to economic development, they were referred to as 'underdeveloped' or 'developing' countries. Meanwhile, gross national product (GNP) was used for purposes of comparing the economic status of nations and gross domestic product (GDP) for comparing levels of development. More recently, the World Bank introduced a system of categorizing countries on the basis of gross national income per capita (GNI) for comparing differing needs for economic development, and this classification has caught on more generally for categorizing countries into low-, middle- and high-income countries with some in-betweens. In general, what are called developing countries fall into the combined category called 'low-and middle-income' countries (LMICs). The latest statistics for this GNI classification is given by the World Bank (2013). In this book, I refer almost interchangeably (although with slight differences of nuance) to 'Third World', 'developing' or 'underdeveloped' countries, and 'Global South'; and correspondingly I refer to the 'West', 'developed countries' and 'Global North'. Also, I refer to the first group as LMICs and the second group as high-income countries (HICs). And, very occasionally I refer to the 'Rest' as the opposite of the 'West' and once or twice I use the term 'Majority World' as an alternative to Global South.

In my earlier books, for example, in the second edition of *Mental Health, Race and Culture* (Fernando, 2002), I highlighted cultural differences in traditions by comparing 'West' and 'East', equivalent to the West–the Rest dichotomy. Sometimes, I presented the East–West dichotomy as a 'traditional–modern' dichotomy, although what is traditional and what is modern is a moot point, considering that modern science seems more in line theoretically with ancient Indian understanding of the human condition (vis-à-vis the psyche) than with those of twentieth-century 'western' viewpoints (Capra, 1982). In the third edition (Fernando, 2010), the East–West model had already lost some of its relevance. As Pieterse (2009) points out, a result of complex cultural changes in the first decade of the twenty-first century is that cultural *hybridity*, rather than cultural *difference*, has become a leading paradigm in social science and cultural studies. However, in the second decade (the present), it is becoming apparent that power games sometimes backed by military force are being played out using implied cultural superiority of so-called western values, standards and ethics (over those of 'the other' or more specifically the Third World). And, as Homi Bhabha (1994) says, there is 'a kinship between the normative paradigms of colonial anthropology [with its inherent racism] and the contemporary discourse of aid and development agencies' (1994, p. 242). Human rights are much talked about, but 'humanitarianism' is often used cynically for imperial purposes (Bricmont, 2007). It is in this context that cultural systems (including psychology and psychiatry) are being imposed and this imposition is sometimes called 'globalization' (see Chapter 1). So trying to understand what is happening in the field of 'culture'—differences, similarities and, most importantly, hybridity and change—comparing West and East or the West and the Rest still hold some relevance, although the protagonists (as it were) are now usually referred to as 'North' and 'South' or 'Global North' and 'Global South' or, when emphasizing the fact that most people live in the latter, 'Minority World' and 'Majority World'.

In the latter parts of this book, I refer to not-for-profit organizations that carry out much development work in the Global South. They are referred to loosely as non-governmental organizations (NGOs) or INGOs ('I' for 'international') when their activities extend to several countries. The terminology goes back to the time when the United Nations (UN) got going after the end of WWII. Two types of organizations were created to have a relationship with the UN (Willetts, 2013): global intergovernmental organizations and INGOs. The latter are recognized by the UN and are eligible to have 'consultative status' with UN bodies: 'They operate like pressure groups in British and American politics, except that they have greater participation rights in the UN than pressure groups have in the House of Commons or Congress' (Willetts, 2013, p. 6). Apart from these UN-accredited bodies, various other not-for-profit bodies active in the LMICs tend to call themselves NGOs. Most of the funding of both the accredited and non-accredited NGOs usually come from private bodies (trusts) or governments in the Global North, but it is important to note that locally controlled NGOs (also called community organizations) have considerably more authentic representatives of local people than do the INGOs with UN accreditation and NGOs that are controlled by organizations or governments in HICs.

Finally, a word about the pharmaceutical industry which is composed of many profit-making (often multinational) companies controlled in the Global North. I sometimes shorten this to 'Pharma' and occasionally to 'Big Pharma' to emphasize 'its extraordinary wealth ... [which can be] gleaned by the sheer scale of its operations, not just geographically across the globe but by any standard economic terms of reference— revenues, sales teams, profits, growths' (Law, 2006, p. 28). The role that Pharma plays in mental health development in the Global South, and how much it influences mental health policy generally, is difficult to evaluate. Critical commentaries on Pharma's ways of operating in the health sector in the Global North have been covered in books such as *The Truth about Drug Companies* (Angell, 2005), *Big Pharma* (Law, 2006) and *Bad Pharma* (Goldacre, 2012). An important point to note is that the loyalty of Pharma is inevitably to shareholders of the individual companies.

Outline of the book

The book is in four parts. Part I, 'Cultural History of Madness, Psychiatry and Mental Health' (Chapters 1, 2 and 3); Part II, 'What Happened in the Majority World' (Chapters 4 and 5); Part III, 'Psychiatry and Mental Health after the Second World War: Exporting Psychiatry to the Global

South' (Chapters 6, 7 and 8); and Part IV, 'Developing Mental Health Services' (Chapters 9, 10 and 11).

Parts

Part I sets the stage for subsequent parts. After a brief discussion of culture and globalization, it traces the rise of psychiatry and psychology in the West, associated with its post-Enlightenment take on madness and the 'mind'. While the illness approach to many human problems dominated thinking in the Global North, leading to the search for medical remedies for curing illness, this tradition contrasted with (non-western) traditions in the rest of the world, covering similar fields. Further, misperceptions of the 'other' resulted in the West being pitted against the Rest and rejecting knowledge and wisdom of non-western cultures. Part II describes the situation in many parts of the (culturally) non-western world until about the mid-twentieth century vis-à-vis the likely experience of people who may have had (in psychiatric terms) mental health problems and mental illness. It examines what is known about the ways in which problems and illness seen (in western cultural idioms) as 'mental' were viewed in the non-western world and what help (or services) may have been available if needed. Also, it describes the impact of colonial psychiatry, focusing on its effect on ordinary people of the Third World. Part III looks at the changes across the globe over the past six decades in what may be called the 'mental health scene'. This part of the book analyses some of the social and economic forces active in spreading psychiatry worldwide and examines how professionals and other individuals on both sides of the North–South divide are drawn into powerful systems associated with multinational corporations (MNCs) that promote the adoption of bio-medical psychiatry across the world. Part IV outlines some changes in mental health services in the Global North that could be instituted without too much upheaval and then proposes ways of developing mental health and well-being services in the Global South in an ethical and sustainable manner, suited to the needs of the people concerned. The ultimate requirement in both North and South is for services to be derived from *local* thinking, developed bottom-up and home-grown. Afterthoughts at the end of the book focus briefly and tentatively on the future of psychiatry and mental health service provision in general.

Chapters

Chapter 1 ('Culture and globalization in relation to mental health') is an introductory essay discussing the meaning of culture worldwide and ideas about globalization that have recently come to the fore. Chapter 2 ('Understanding madness, mental illness and mental health') traces the way discourses around these topics arose historically in western culture; how post-Enlightenment thinking in Europe led to a system of knowledge subsumed in the disciplines of Euro-American psychiatry and western psychology; and how the western tradition about mental illness and mental health emerged as a system of medicalized psychiatry and biologized psychology. Then, this western cultural tradition is compared to non-western traditions covering related matters by exploring what we know about thinking in Indian and Chinese medicine and various spiritual and religious beliefs that informed these traditions. Chapter 3 ('Medicalization of human problems in the West') describes the main social and political forces that played out in the West resulting in constructing the (western) illness model for a variety of human experiences and behaviours.

Although it is difficult to set mental health and ill-health in non-western cultural settings in a proper historical context because the language (of mental health and illness and allied concepts) derive from thinking in European culture, Chapter 4 ('Mental health and mental illness in non-western countries') has a go at presenting the background to mental health in the Third World drawing out deductions on what appears to have gone on in Asia, Africa and pre-Columbian America in the case of people who today (under the influence of psychiatric thinking) may be designated as 'mentally ill' or suffering from 'mental health problems'. Chapter 5 ('Colonial psychiatry') describes briefly what is known of the western-style asylums installed (occasionally with other psychiatric services) in Asian and African colonies, with little concern as to their suitability or acceptance locally. It is questionable as to what extent they were used by local people as places for treatment or care but they have left a legacy that is a burden on LMICs. Also, so-called observations by colonial psychiatrists contributed to the 'knowledge' that fed into psychiatry and became problematic for immigrants of Asian and African descent that settled in the West after de-colonization.

Chapter 6 ('Medication revolution and emerging discontents') sets out the changes that occurred in psychiatry as drug therapy for 'mental illness' came on the scene in the 1970s. The scope of what was defined as 'mental illness' massively expanded, and the modern brand of drug-based bio-medical psychiatry emerged in western Europe and North America. The chapter outlines the serious problems with Euro-American bio-medical psychiatry that are now being critically examined. Chapter 7 ('Ethnic problems in the West and neo-imperialism abroad') considers the scene in the late 1970s and 1980s when psychiatry was seen as not fit for purpose in the case of many ethnic minorities of Asian and African backgrounds living in UK and as part of a system of control of African-Americans in the USA and black people in Europe. The chapter explores how this situation resonated with psychiatry being pushed on to LMICs in spite of its apparent unsuitability—psychiatric imperialism. Chapter 8 ('International politics of mental health and psychiatry') discusses events in the era of globalization seen in a context of western power and neo-liberal policies being adopted in many countries worldwide. The role of the World Health Organization and the movement for 'global' mental health are critically examined, and some deductions are made as to the forces driving the imposition of psychiatric models of diagnosis in LMICs in association with marketing of psychotropic drugs.

Chapter 9 ('Modernizing mental health services in the Global North') formulates practical changes that could improve services in the UK and have more general applicability in the Global North. Chapter 10 ('Mental health and well-being in the Global South') suggests that the primary need in the Global South is for political action to address social determinants of health and that development of ground-level services should be ethical and sustainable while ensuring consistency with local cultures. The approach in developing mental health and well-being services in the Global South should be one that promotes a bottom-up approach so that the final products are home-grown and owned by the people of the countries concerned. Finally, Chapter 11 ('Afterthoughts: Power, diagnosis and the Majority World') presents some thoughts about the future of psychiatry in mental health services across the world; discusses the uncertainties that are currently prevalent in the field of development; and reiterates a call for ethical development of services for mental health and well-being in LMICs, where, compared to the Global North, the vast majority of people are poor, voiceless and remain culturally 'non-western' in many ways, with very different ideas about what mental health means and very different needs and wants when compared to most people in the rich western countries.

Part I

Cultural History of Madness, Psychiatry and Mental Health

After a discussion of culture and globalization, this first part of the book traces the rise of psychiatry and the discourse on 'mental health' in the western world, associated with its post-Enlightenment approach to madness and the 'mind'. While the illness approach to many human problems came to dominate thinking in the Global North leading to the search for medical remedies directed at curing illness, misperceptions of the 'other' resulted in the West being pitted against the Rest.

Part I

Cultural History of Madness, Psychiatry and Mental Health

1
Culture and Globalization in Relation to Mental Health

People all over the world are implicated in individual problems of living, interacting with one another and the environment, trying to understand the purpose of our lives, working out in practice how we get along with one another and, finally, dealing with the end of life as individuals. We tend to address these issues not only in concert with others, as communities and societies, but also as individuals. However we think of ourselves at any particular moment, we are all biological, social and spiritual beings, essentially the same. In that sense, we are *global* people. But over the centuries of our existence as human beings, groups of people as communities, nations and families have developed ways of negotiating their journeys through life, relating to whatever environment they find themselves in and changing aspects of it to suit their needs, and dealing with problems (though not necessarily overcoming them). And these ways became set into traditional ways of behaviour, belief, world-views and so on—they became 'cultures'. And now we hear a lot about 'globalization' without any clear definition of the term or a consistent understanding of what it means (see below). The purpose of this chapter is to explore briefly the connection between culture—more specifically cultural diversity—across the world and the diverse meanings attached to globalization in relation to mental health and mental health services. The diverse meanings of mental health worldwide are not discussed in this chapter. Exploration of this topic runs through a good part of the rest of the book, especially in Chapters 2 and 4.

Nature of culture

Cultures were regarded at one time in the English-language literature as relatively fixed, dependent on learning and essentially territorial;

localized often to one part of the world, forming the culture of a society or group of people. But 'culture' is now understood and written about somewhat differently. The notion of culture goes back to nineteenth-century romanticism and was elaborated in twentieth-century anthropology (Pieterse, 1995) which talked of 'shared patterns of belief, feeling and adaptation which people carry in their minds' (Leighton and Hughes, 1961, p. 447). But this idea of culture as 'a unique way of life' first took hold in anthropology during colonialism in order to separate the colonizing West from (what the West saw as) 'uncivilized' people that were being colonized (Eagleton, 2000, p. 26) and so it could not last. What has emerged after de-colonization, and more so in the post-modern terrain of the late twentieth century going into the twenty-first, is the notion of culture as something that is malleable and changeable; it depends not just on traditions that people inherit but also on historical and political influences in a context of power relations at various levels and at various times. Homi Bhabha's (1994) *Location of Culture* emphasizes the hybridity of cultural forms and the ways in which racism, most evident during colonialism and slavery, is closely involved in the manifestation of cultural diversity, especially in many parts of the western world; and Edward Said's (1994) *Culture and Imperialism* unravels the intimate connections between understandings of culture presented in Anglo-American literature and European domination of the rest of the world since about the late sixteenth century. Whether referring to that of an individual or a group, culture is now seen as something that is dynamic and far from static—a flexible system of values and worldviews that people live by, and through which they define identities and negotiate their lives (for fuller discussion, see Fernando, 2010).

While the term 'culture' is still applied to an individual person or group—and this is the main use of the term in the field of mental health—the term is now used for a broad range of situations associated with people and/or institutions, quite apart from its rather elitist use in some circles when some people are described as 'cultured' meaning more sophisticated than other uncultured or less-cultured people. In the mental health field, we talk now of family cultures, or cultures of whole communities in addition to the culture of an individual. When we say that a society is 'multicultural', we imply that there are broad cultural differences between groups of people within the society. We also refer to cultures of professional groups, for example, 'medical culture', 'police culture', or institutions or systems such as a particular hospital or the health service or the system of psychiatry or clinical psychology. In fact, seemingly involved in so many fields of discourse and literature, the term 'culture' is fast becoming an easy explanation for almost any activity associated with human beings and the ways in which institutions and systems consisting of several individuals function.

Although there is a perception that cultures of people ('culture' used in its limited sense) have in some way remained 'pure' until modern times, in actual fact, cultural interchanges and cultural mingling have always taken place—at times very extensively, resulting in mixtures seen as 'new' cultures or termed (sometimes pejoratively) 'creole' or hybrid cultures. Historian J. J. Clarke (1997) points out that 'commercial and cultural intercourse between East and West was well established at the time when philosophical foundations of western thought were being laid down in Greece' (p. 37), and that it continued along the silk routes between the Mediterranean and the East. The direct links between Europe and the East were curtailed by the imposition of the Islamic empire (see Chapter 2) but resumed after the thirteenth century as illustrated by European travellers to China, such as Marco Polo. This mixing of cultures has been greatly accelerated by better communication, easier travel and increased migration across the world during the past four or five decades.

The discourse on 'culture' that is applicable to mental health mainly concerns the culture of the individual because of the emphasis on the individual in the (western) interpretation of 'mental health' (see Chapter 2). But even here it is recognized that individual culture rests on a bed of traditional family culture, the culture of the community they are part of, the wider body of people they felt attached to, the region(s) they live in and even perhaps the 'imagined communities' (Anderson, 1991, title page) they are connected to. These ramifications of culture determine to a large extent people's behaviour, and more generally, their social systems, religious systems and beliefs, worldviews and, most important of all (for the purposes of this book), their concept of the human condition, the meaning of life itself. In other words, 'traditional culture' forms an important background to a great deal of people's lived experience, how they perceive and make sense of their lives, what they see as natural and so on. It should be pointed out here that (as discussed above) culture is not a fixed entity but subject to almost constant change and so difficult to pin down. And it could be quite complicated and problematic to work out, at any given time, what particular aspects of their traditional culture affect any one person or group ('cultural group'). But differences are always there.

Globalization

Globalization, 'the successor to the debates on modernity and post-modernity in the understanding of sociocultural change' (Featherstone and Lash, 1995, p. 1), has recently become a prominent theme in many fields, even, since about 2010, in the field of mental health (see discussion of global health below). The term 'globalization' frequently implies an underlying message of westernization (of the non-western world) and is often tied up with modernity, a concept 'unproblematically associated with "the West" ' (King, 1995, p. 111), implying that the world is becoming more uniform and standardized through technological, commercial and cultural synchronization emanating from the West (Pieterse, 1995).

In the field of culture, where cultural exchanges and cultural diffusion across the world are inevitable and the fact that human beings are social beings, globalization may be seen as something inevitable when groups of people in communication with each other share ideas, technologies and so on. This could be seen as a natural process—*passive globalization*. A different take on globalization is put forward by Petras and Veltmeyer (2001): To them it represents a movement that imposes systemic change through a variety of institutions becoming 'the new imperialism—the new system of "global governance" ' (pp. 12–13). This could be called *forced globalization* where, in actual fact, the discourse of globalization obfuscates and hides what is really taking place. This neo-imperialism may take the form of western systems (of psychiatric diagnosis, for example) being imposed as a condition of economic aid for supposed modernization of health systems; or more subtly through pressures from evaluation of institutional systems or advice of experts from (western) centres of excellence. The thinking around globalization and culture that I have outlined is summarized in Table 1.1.

Clearly, forced and passive (or natural) globalization either may occur together reinforcing each other (in which case the outcomes are mixed) or may occur in conflict with each other; some aspects of what happens

Table 1.1   Globalization and culture

Passive globalization
Natural process through diffusion of ideas and cultural forms in voluntary
   interchange

Forced globalization
Process imposed overtly—for example, as part of economic aid for
   'modernization'—or subtly, for example, via institutional pressures

---

being natural and some forced, in which case there are winners and losers. In Chapter 10, I suggest that the current globalization discourse in the field of mental health tends to camouflage a process whereby western ideologies and ways of thinking are being imposed in the Third World in order to structure developing countries in such a way that perpetuates western power and profits multinational corporations.

In considering mental health development as a social process, the loose use of the word 'globalization' means that it can mean different things to different people and in different circumstances. Jonathan Friedman (1995) suggests that we could see globalization as something that is limited to the formation of global institutional structures 'that organize the already existing global field and global cultural forms' (p. 75) that may, at most, have an indirect effect on the diverse cultural forms (such as medical and religious systems meant to help people with personal problems, including mental health problems) but, on the whole, allow different systems to flourish. This could be seen as an 'organizational globalization'. Alternatively, we could see globalization as a global force that compresses 'civilizational cultures, national societies, intra- and cross-national movements and organizations, sub-societies and ethnic groups, intra-societal quasi groups, individuals, and so on... [yielding] "third cultures"—such as transnational movements and international organizations' (Robertson, 1992, p. 61). Initially discussed in political and economic terms (of trade treaties and political action) at an international level, globalization would then imply a 'global culture'. In this case, globalization is intrusive and comes up against (that is, in conflict with) existing cultural forms and indeed the pluralism of cultural forms, including healing systems and medical systems that exist in the world. Such an intrusive globalization, inducing, or trying to induce, a *global* culture, opposes the right to be 'different' and, in doing so, impinges on the rights of national or ethnic communities. Given the geopolitical power structures in the world today, this sort of globalization is no different to imperialism and akin to what was described as forced globalization (above). The thinking around globalization and mental health development is shown in Table 1.2.

A point about the popular use of the terms 'global health' and the more recent appearance in the public arena of the term 'global mental health' should be noted here although discussed in more detail in Chapter 8. In short, what was thought of as 'international health' (IH), to refer to the health status of countries outside the West, became, in the mid-1990s, 'global health' mainly to emphasize how human health is interconnected across the globe (McInnes and Lee, 2012). It appears

Table 1.2 Globalization and mental health development

Organizational globalization
Formation of institutional structures to ease cooperation worldwide

Intrusive globalization
Pressures to compress local diversity into global uniformity

---

that the term 'global mental health' came into use after joint directors of a newly formed Centre for Global Mental Health announced it as a 'new global health field [that] comes of age' (Patel and Prince, 2010, p. 1976). The term itself has been described as an 'oxymoron' (Summerfield, 2012, p. 3) because *mental* health (unlike general health whose parameters can be measured) is understood very differently across the world, the meaning given to it being determined largely by cultural background and social context (see Chapter 2). Global perspectives on, or perceptions of, mental health that this book is concerned with are as much about difference as similarity; as much about diversity as concordance; as much about individuals, their societies and their cultures as about the unity of the human race as well as the need for people around the world to recognize their common humanity.

Conclusions

Issues around culture and globalization are implicit throughout this book. The former has a long history in the field of mental health while the latter only recently emerged as a theme in the field of mental health. The use of the term 'culture' in mental health discourse is usually limited to matters to do with individuals (so referring to culture of individuals) and the connections they have to people and events around them as well as their heritage and background—in effect, the total reality within which people live their lives. Globalization of concepts around mental health may either mean that ideas and ways of thinking are being spread across the world more easily than they were in the past through *passive* globalization, which has always taken place but has been greatly accelerated recently because of ease of travel and communication across the world; or else means that particular ways of thinking are being *imposed* so that cultural changes are coming about as a result of economic and political forces—in other words, there is *forced* globalization. When it comes to developing mental health services, the discourse of 'globalization' confuses issues. In this instance, if globalization merely implies improving understanding, and hence cooperation, between local systems and systems in other places, all well and good. But if globalization means that global remedies and global ideas about mental health and illness are to be imposed, the current power structures would predicate pressures to abolish diversity and enforce western ways of thinking and western therapies worldwide—something that is contrary to the human rights of individuals and communities.

The interplay between culture and globalization in the mental health field is complicated by the fact that (a) culture (of an individual or group) is not something that is static but both changeable according to context and malleable in that it is likely to be subjected to various forces that impinge on it; and (b) globalization as an active powerful force (forced globalization) may impose changes, including cultural ones, for economic and political purposes in a context of geopolitical power—something that amounts to a westernization of the non-western world because of the current global power imbalances. However, whatever changes globalization or westernization bring, fundamental differences between peoples in terms of their basic understanding of the human condition, what 'mental' means or does not mean and how they see illness and health, all these are likely to continue because of the very nature of human beings as *cultural* and *social*, in addition to being biological, genetic and so on.

2
Understanding Madness, Mental Illness and Mental Health

The concept of madness is evident in all human cultures and may be as old as mankind itself (Porter, 2002). However, the talk of mental illness and mental health is relatively recent. Every cultural tradition includes a concept of illness (McQueen, 1978), and often of health meaning freedom from illness, but what illness means and what health means vary across cultures. However, *concern* with illness is universal (White, 1982), and illness is usually dealt with by medical systems, systems of healing and so on. Nevertheless, the medical system in a cultural tradition may overlap in many ways with its religious system or other aspects of society; and the concepts of mind and of matters to do with 'mental activity' have generally become entangled with issues about health and illness. Notions around madness, illness/health and the mind that emerged in the post-Enlightenment culture of Europe in the seventeenth century spread from there to North America and other regions where European settlement occurred, finally crystallizing during the eighteenth and nineteenth centuries in a western tradition evident most forcibly in (western) psychiatry. And these ideas, and even the practice of psychiatry, have spread, although so far to a limited extent, in the non-western world too.

In this chapter, I examine briefly the ideologies, and beliefs appertaining to (what we today call) 'mental health' and its connections to (what we call today) mental ill-health (or mental disorder/illness) that developed in both western and non-western regions of the world, and how these became relatively fixed, forming the background to ways of thinking about human beings in general. I shall refer to these as 'traditional cultures' or more briefly as 'traditions', rather than 'cultures', mainly because 'cultures' are no longer seen as fixed entities (see Chapter 1). Fuller discussions of the material in this chapter are available in the second and third editions of *Mental Health, Race and Culture* (Fernando, 2002, 2010), while some classic studies are available in books on transcultural psychiatry such as *Ethnopsychiatry* edited by Gaines (1992) and *Culture and Depression* edited by Kleinman and Good (1985a).

For convenience in organizing this chapter, I take as a starting point the European (that became the Euro-American) tradition of what constitutes 'madness' (insanity), and how this was elaborated and added to in evolving a western tradition of mental health and mental illness articulated largely through Euro-American psychiatry. It is convenient to do so because much more information is available about the way knowledge about madness, mental health and mental illness developed in the West compared to what we know about the genesis of similar ideas in other places. Then, using that 'western' model for comparison, I look at the traditions of non-western cultures in terms of similarities and differences: How ideas about 'mental' or psychological health and ill-health (or illness) that are cross-culturally equivalent to those elaborated in the West were envisaged and understood in different regions of the world; and what ideas developed there about the nature of the human mind reflected in concepts of health and illness. For the sake of simplicity, I shall refer to regions of the world where stable civilizations developed with recognizable and documented social systems, although acknowledging that these did not develop in isolation from each other nor did they take a clearly recognizable unitary form. I admit that readers may see it as unnatural to lump together various individual traditions as either 'western' or 'non-western'. But I suggest that this approach is the most useful way of generalizing concisely the cultural diversity of different ways of understanding mental health and illness developed across the world (a matter discussed briefly as points about language in 'Introduction'). I acknowledge, however, that cultures have intermingled and traditions have not remained static. Today's world is characterized by cultural mixtures—hybrid cultures—with the reality of cultural diasporas and ethnic groups scattered across the world, interconnected with each other and, at the same time, interacting with each other in multiple ways (Pieterse, 2007).

The traditions originating in non-western cultures would have reflected the ways in which people designated (in a western tradition) as suffering from mental health problems or mental illness/disorder were regarded in regions of the world that were outside the West. Also, we need to take on board the fact that these traditions, to some extent at least, travelled with people when they migrated or were forcibly taken away from their native habitat, and they persist to a greater or lesser extent in ethnic or cultural diasporas in the West. For example, some aspects of their original culture persist in Indian or African diasporas in North America, although, in the latter case, much of their original African culture may have become distorted or suppressed by the effects of slavery and subsequent oppressions. In fact, the transfer of culture with migration would always be subject to many social and political processes and is never complete. Further, as time goes on after migration, emergent cultures (and traditions) develop. For example, originally African people who had settled in the Caribbean (having been forcibly relocated) developed a specifically 'Caribbean' culture; and then black Caribbean people who migrated to the UK developed, in a context of British racism, a (British) 'West Indian culture' of the 1970s (Hall *et al.*, 1978, p. 350), becoming one of the 'new [British] ethnicities' of the 1990s (Cohen, 1999, p. 5; Hall, 1992, p. 252).

Western tradition

The changes in European thinking during the (European) Enlightenment of the seventeenth and eighteenth centuries resulted in positivist ideas that became embodied in how mental health and mental illness (the disordered mind) came to be seen. But some of the ideas can be traced to thinking about medical illness developed in the Hippocratic tradition of ancient Greece, elaborated in Arabic medicine of the tenth to thirteenth centuries (see below). Out of the study of madness (interpreted as resulting from disturbed mind) emerged (western) psychology—the study of the 'normal' mind and the concept of 'mental health' (healthy mind).

In his foreword to the first English translation of Foucault's *History of Madness*, Jean Khalfa (2006) makes the fundamental point 'that whether madness is described as a religious or philosophical phenomenon (an experience or inspiration, loss of mind, etc.), or an objective medical essence (as in classifications of madness developed by psychiatry), these conceptions [of madness] are not discoveries but historical constructions of meaning'; hence, the medicalization of madness 'tells us about what must have changed in society as a whole for such a transformation to occur' (2006, pp. xiv–xv). Foucault (2006) points out that unreason as something *positive* was identified (in Europe) as the characteristic of madness during the fourteenth to sixteenth centuries; it was only later that unreason was seen as pathological and madness as 'illness':

There is a tendency to believe that the mad were individuated as a result of a process of medical humanitarianism, as if the figure of their individuality was never anything other than pathological. In fact, in the Middle Ages [in Europe] long before the medical status that came with positivism, the mad had already acquired a sort of personal density, although more as character types than pathological cases. (1960, pp. 116–17)

Medicalization of madness

Prior to the (European) Enlightenment, also called the 'Age of Reason' (Barzun, 2000, p. 314; Smith, 2008, p. 139), madness was seen as the state of mind of people who had lost their 'reason' or did not possess it to start with—people characterized by unreason. Then came the creation of social institutions for the confinement of 'the mad' (the insane), which gathered pace in the eighteenth century. The underlying agenda for creating them was ethical and political whereby the mad (ostensibly for their own good), together with other socially undesirable people, were excluded from society. Being locked up, they ('the mad') became the object of study and observation, and madness or lunacy increasingly became seen as disease. And so, the concept of unreason as a positive state, and not just as the lack of reason, gradually lost its significance. By end of the eighteenth century, institutions devoted to the 'care' of the mad were in full flood; and, in the next century, the lunatic asylum became the mental hospital where the need to 'cure' went hand in hand with protecting society: 'The mad are now [eighteenth century] locked up in *order to be cured*' (Khalfa, 2006, p. xviii, emphasis in original). As medical people were put in charge of these asylums/hospitals, madness was seen as an affliction of the brain just as various other diseases were afflictions of other organs of the body. Madness as illness was then something separate from the 'mad' person, to be dealt with *positively*.

Medical doctors who treated madness, or 'mental alienation' as it was called sometimes, were initially called 'mad doctors' or alienists (Shorter, 1997, p. 17). As they grappled with madness as mental illness, they established power over the mentally ill and also made it possible for the 'appearance of a psychology [of mental illness]...a cultural fact peculiar to the Western world since the nineteenth century' (Foucault, 2006, p. 529). In other words, the (western) study of the mind—'psychology', promoted in modern times as a 'scientific' discipline—came about through study of madness. As Foucault (2006) puts it: '*[H]omo psychologicus* (psychological man) is descended from *homo mente captus* (insane man)' (2006, p. 529). Since then, (western) psychology and psychiatry have led the thinking around madness, mental illness and mental health—at first in the West but gradually all over the world—but only up to a point in many places (see Chapters 4, 5 and 7). To Foucault, '[western] psychology is always, by its very nature, at a crossroads...between the subject and the object, between within and without, between lived experience and knowledge' (2006, pp. 529–30). And psychiatry clings to its illness model to describe increasingly diverse types of lived experience, beliefs and behaviour.

Biologization of the mind

In the latter part of the nineteenth century, psychology (in the West) became progressively more biological under the influence of Darwinism (Murphy, 1938) and the mind was increasingly seen as something biological. Hereditary factors were quoted for nearly every individual or group variation or difference in behaviour, thinking and so on, all seen against a background of evolutionary advantage and survival of the fittest. Meanwhile, psychiatry structured mental illnesses as circumscribed entities explicable in natural, usually physical, terms. And with western psychology espousing eugenics, 'the science which deals with...inborn qualities of race' (Galton, 1904, p. 1), mental illness was attributed to inherited defects that could not be corrected, tying in with the concept of 'degeneration' enunciated by a medical doctor, Bénédict-Auguste Morel (1857). According to Pick (1989), who studied the derivation of the idea of degeneration in some depth, Morel 'was pre-occupied by the seemingly remorseless rise in the numbers of the insane and the apparent inability of mental medicine to cure its patients' (1989, p. 54). Morel postulated degeneration as a deviation from normality recognizable by physical stigmata that resulted inevitably in moral and intellectual collapse of an individual; he also suggested that doctors should not concern themselves in cure of lunatics but in merely containing them so that they do not contaminate society. Helped by the developing science of genetics, this led to assumptions of madness being inherited and incurable. In fact, by the 1920s, mental illness was firmly established as a genetic problem, the (then) recently named 'schizophrenia' (see Chapter 3) being the epitome of genetic illness of the mind. By the middle of the twentieth century, all mental disorders were viewed as inborn conditions, which *ipso facto* (at that time) were not amenable to treatment.

As psychiatry and (western) psychology gained power and influence in Europe and North America, the practices in its application changed but the tradition set in the eighteenth century, with its basic tenets about mental health and mental illness, remained the same. The search for understanding 'unreason' (the original characteristic of madness) had all but disappeared by the early twentieth century, except for parts of Freudian psychoanalysis that 'raised the possibility of a dialogue with unreason' within a medical framework (Foucault, 2006, p. 339). Cartesian duality remained a fundamental part of the psychiatric paradigm: On a canvass of the mind seen as either a mere function of the brain or an entity independent of the brain but, in some way, related to it; psychiatry designated mental illness in terms of diagnoses, ignoring the fact that there were no objective criteria by which to identify them (for discussion of this topic, see Bentall, 2010).

West/non-West differences

In most non-western cultural traditions, including those of pre-Columbian America, the conceptualization of mind and body and ideas about illness and health developed very differently to that in the West. A major problem is that a reliable body of information on the background and traditions of Africa and pre-Columbian America is not available for several reasons: In the case of Africa, the subject is vast and relatively unresearched (Karenga, 1982). Also, in most parts of Africa, sources of history were 'griots, a class of professional oral historians... [who held]... the collective memory of an ethnic group, nation or empire' (ibid, p. 53)—a vulnerable form of record keeping; and European conquests led to the loss of information about African societies before slavery and colonization, as well as to the distortion of history to fit into racist models of African 'primitiveness'. In the case of South America, the wanton destruction by the Spanish conquerors that followed Columbus resulted in genocide, plunder and cultural pillage, all but destroying the civilizations in the region that preceded European conquest. In North America, aggressive colonization by Europeans left the indigenous people restricted to live in reservations, and their children often being forcibly Europeanized in 'residential schools' (Haig-Brown, 1988).

We should note here that Asian and African psychologies (as study of the individual mind) are very different in fundamental ways to western psychology: The latter came about through a study of madness while the non-western psychologies came out of spirituality and personal introspection. The notion attributed to Descartes (Cartesian doctrine) that has dominated western thinking about human beings since the mid-seventeenth century (see Capra, 1982) states that the body is governed by mechanical laws but the mind (or soul) is free and immortal, so that a person 'lives through two collateral histories' (Ryle, 1990, p. 13). And then, as western psychology developed in the late eighteenth century, it was influenced by studies of the nervous system, especially reports of correlations between mental activity and brain structure, and by various other theories apparently supporting a mechanistic basis for mental activities. Western psychology imitated methods of the 'pure sciences' (physics and chemistry), supplanting introspection by systematized judgements made seemingly objective by converting them into numerical presentations (quantification). Most non-western psychologies are holistic in taking on the whole individual rather than the individual mind divided into parts, as emotions, cognitions and so on. Not only are their roots very different (see above), non-western psychologies being embedded in religion and philosophy and western psychology in science (or whatever went as 'science'), but western psychology was applied in a secular, or even anti-religious, context. The (European) Enlightenment that gave rise to psychology had pushed religion into a corner so that anything spiritual was excluded from psychology as well as (to a large extent) from politics, philosophy and even morality. In non-western traditions, religion and philosophy are jointly integrated into all aspects of knowledge in a way it is not in the West. In eastern traditions, rationality is seen as *maya*, illusory and superficial. Chinese philosophy, at least the non-Confucian variety, sees reality, whose ultimate essence is called *tao*, as a process of continual flow and change. Safaya (1976) writes that 'mind' in Indian psychology is an organ of action, not just of thinking; and consciousness is vested in the 'self', not in mind or body. And both Indian and Chinese traditions have strong ethical components.

Illness experience

An overarching way in which western tradition differs from others is evident in the way it handles the *experience* of mental health and illness. In non-western holistic traditions, subjective and objective experiences are so intertwined and interposed one into the other that they cannot be separated. But a traditional western non-holistic approach would attribute ill-health to either an external cause or an internal one, each seen as a separate entity. A holistic tradition promotes a sense of health

Table 2.1   Influence of holism on health and illness

	Cultural tradition	
	Holistic	Non-holistic
External (objective) vs. internal (subjective) experience	Intertwined and interposed within each other	Distinct and separate from each other
Causation of ill-health	Experienced as both internal and external *at the same time*	Experienced as either external or internal, one impacting on the other
Experience of health	Harmonious balance between different aspects of self and environment	Subjective well-being distinct from external influences

Source: Slightly adapted from Fernando (2010).

as a harmonious balance between various forces in the person and/or social context as opposed to seeing health as an individualized sense of well-being. All this is summarized in Table 2.1 reproduced with slight changes from an earlier publication (Fernando, 2010, p. 42).

Many practical differences appertaining to the individual flow from all this: In non-western traditions, a person's external and internal experiences are not just related to each other but they are *one and the same*; and experience is both subjective and objective *at the same time*, nothing is separate from anything else. The *yin/yang* terminology of Chinese tradition represents such a view. In looking for an analogy in the western tradition, the closest one can get is systems theory 'which looks at the world in terms of the interrelatedness and interdependence of all phenomena, and in this framework an integrated whole whose properties cannot be reduced to those of its parts' (Capra, 1982, p. 26). Helen Graham (1986), in a review of the cultural context of humanist psychology, writes: 'Eastern culture, in its concern with intangibles rather than "facts", with emotionality rather than rationality, gives pre-eminence to the subjective and experiential' (1986, p. 5). Contrasting the activity of introspection in western culture with that of its counterpart in the Indian tradition, Sudhir Kakar (1984), an Indian psychotherapist trained in the West but deeply immersed in Indian traditions and practising in India, notes that, in the former, definitions of self and identity are contingent upon 'examining, sorting out and scrutinizing' one's own life, while in meditative (Indian) procedures of 'self-realization', introspection dwells on the 'self' of Indian philosophy 'uncontaminated by time and space' (1984, p. 7). Nobles (1986) notes, 'unlike the mathematical illusion of normality found in the West, normality which would be consistent with African thought is a normal which is equivalent to one's nature' (1986, p. 112).

Concepts of health and illness

In simple shorthand, eastern traditions see health as a harmonious balance between various forces in the person and the social context, while western traditions see health as individualized sense of well-being. In traditional Chinese way of thinking, illness is an imbalance of *yin* and *yang* (two complementary poles of life energy), to be corrected by attempts to re-establish 'balance' (Aakster, 1986; Kaptchuk, 2000; Wu, 1984), a concept that is not easily grasped intellectually by a western-educated person. Those aspects of a human being that western psychology would call 'emotions' are integral parts of all sickness although reified 'emotional diseases' are not recognized (Wu, 1984). Hammer (2000) sees 'balance' (that Chinese doctors aim to achieve in dealing with illness) as not something to be achieved 'since there are two opposite constructs around the issue of balance; one which extols it the other which abhors it, and both of which are necessary' (p. 96). Mental energy is one of five functional energies that form (what in western psychology and medicine would correspond to) the nervous system; and the symbol (representing a word in English) for heart, namely *xin*, is the same as that for mind in Chinese language (Kaptchuk, 2000).

The Indian tradition emphasizes the harmony between the person and his/her group as indicative of health (Kakar, 1984). The human personality in Hindu psychology is the product of a pure Spirit (*Purusa*) and Matter (*Prakriti*); the constituents of western idea of 'mind' are contained in the latter. It is from their interaction that ego-consciousness, self-consciousness, intelligence and other aspects of western mind develop (Safaya, 1976). According to Obeyesekere (1977), the functions of mind in classical Ayurveda (the main medical system in the Indian tradition) resemble the ego-functions of psychoanalytic theory, but, unlike the case of this theory, 'symptoms of psychopathology are due to malfunctioning of the mind, so that Ayurveda would argue that emotional conflicts such as the oedipal ones are not the cause but rather the result of mental malfunction' (p. 157).

Thus, both Chinese and Indian medicine give some importance to altering the way the 'mind' works—'psychotherapy', one may call it.

As for classifications (in the style of western psychiatric diagnoses), using diagnoses is not an appropriate approach for medical systems that are holistic. But ways of analysing and understanding psychological (or psychic) stress or problems that could be seen as 'mental' (in western terms) are found in abundance in Chinese, Indian and most non-western traditions. With respect to India, Kakar (1984) points out that 'Indians have long been involved in constructing explanatory systems for psychic distress and evolving techniques for its alleviation' as exemplified by work of

> the *vaids* of the Hindu Ayurveda and the Siddha systems and the hakim of the Islamic *unani* tradition ... palmists, horoscope specialists, herbalists, diviners, sorcerers and a variety of shamans ... *sadhus,* swamis, *maharajs, babas, matas,* and *bhagwans,* who trace their lineage, in some fashion or other, to the mystical-spiritual traditions of Indian antiquity ... aiming for ... 'soul health'—the restoration of moral and spiritual well-being. (pp. 3–4)

The African tradition conceptualizes health as more social than biological (Lambo, 1964), and deviation from health is embedded 'in traditional magico-religious or spiritual explanation of illness' (Lambo, 1969, p. 201). In African religions, 'no line is drawn between the spiritual and physical' (Mbiti, 1989, p. 5). The connections between African cultures and that of ancient Egypt via the Kemites has been brought together in *Kemet and the African Worldview* edited by Karenga and Carruthers (1962). The thinking of ancient Egypt (Kemet) gave pre-eminence to the notion of soul or spirit; 'the Ka was the divine spirit which endowed all things and which survived past the physical life of the individual'; and psychology in African traditions is the study of the soul (Nobles, 1986, p. 110).

Medical approach

It should be noted that it is not only Europe that has a medical tradition, that is, a tradition of seeing some human problems in terms of personal illness. Medicalization of human problems has occurred in non-western traditions too; the difference is basically in the way medicalization took place, coupled with the scope of what 'medicine' was supposed to cover. Clearly, medical traditions are themselves complex and may well have drawn from each other over the years. A simplified account of some basic cultural differences between them are shown in Table 2.2.

Table 2.2 Medicalization across cultural traditions

Model	Location of illness	Causation of illness	Illness and patient
Western medicine	Mind or body Individual	Genetic–bio-medical Natural events	Separate
Greek medicine	Mind plus body Individual	Humoral	Integrated
Islamic medicine	Mind plus body Individual	Humoral-biological Blended with spirituality and external influences	Partly integrated
Indian medicine	Mind–body– spirit Holistic	Humoral imbalance Spiritual influence	Integrated

Source: Adapted from Fernando (2010).

In western medicine, the Cartesian doctrine ensures that illness is located either in the mind or in the body. In the case of mental illness, causation is seen as genetic-biological as well as being dependent on external natural events, but anything to do with spirituality or the supernatural are excluded. A positivist approach ensures that the 'illness' is objectified as something outside the person with a life of its own. And like other illnesses, mental illness is something separate from the patient; therefore, each illness, usually represented by a diagnosis, has its own history and is distinct from and little to do with the person who is ill. Doctors trained in western medicine speak of the natural history of an illness as something apart from the patient suffering it. Non-western concepts of illness too sometimes recognized a medical dimension that could be objectified, but this objectification did not take over the illness completely; illness still remained an integral part of the individual person, sometimes connected with the world around him or her.

The Greek tradition of medicine located illness in both mind and body with humours circulating in the individual person being the cause of any illness, including those recognized as largely 'mental'. A definite medical approach to madness was evident in the practices within the *māristāns* (Islamic hospitals) of the medieval period (tenth to thirteenth centuries), referred to in Chapter 3. The underlying theme for illness was humoral (from Greek medicine), but once Greek ideas were elaborated in Arabic compendia describing mental illness (Dols, 1992), pressures from events external to the patient (such as supernatural forces or noxious substances such as alcohol) were also seen as playing some part in the aetiology of mental illness. If we look closely at what happened, it is not clear how 'medical' (from a western standpoint of biological illness) the treatment was in the *māristāns*. Foucault (2006) states that, unlike in European institutes of the times, 'a sort of spiritual therapy was carried out, involving music, dance, and theatrical spectacles and readings of marvellous stories' (p. 117). To a very limited extent, this tradition continues in *unani* medicine of India brought there by the Mughals (Masood, 2009). Was it then a medical approach to mental illness that pervaded the *māristāns* or a religious one (based on Islam) or non-religious secular approach—or both or neither? According to Graham (1967) Islamic medicine encapsulated 'a blissful union of science and religion' (p. 47). Dols (1992), whose work provides the most extensive descriptions of how the mental care system worked in the *māristāns*, saw the thinking about madness in Islamic hospitals as a mixture of Galenic (Greek) concepts (such as the humours) blending with pre-Islamic folk medicine and the overarching principle of 'divine causation' (p. 248).

It would seem that spirituality, medicine and the arts, and perhaps much else, all came together in a holistic approach to madness in the Islamic empire. Unfortunately, much of the teaching on mental illness within Islamic medicine has been lost and certainly did not seem to have had much influence on the psychiatry that developed in post-Enlightenment Europe (see section 'Medicalization of Madness'). It is a pity that 'by the late nineteenth century, most of the North African *māristāns* had abandoned their therapeutic functions and merely served as decrepit housing for the mentally ill', even worse than asylums in Europe (Chapter 5). In fact, when the French colonized the Maghreb in the late nineteenth century, the *māristāns* were singled out 'as characteristic of the brutality [sic] and decline of Muslim civilization', to justify alleged civilizing mission of the French (Keller, 2007a, p. 26).

It is possible that the Islamic rulers of India between the sixteenth and nineteenth centuries, the Mughals, introduced the medical approach to madness developed in the *māristāns* (see earlier in this section) to at least a few of the hospitals they built in India (Fabrega, 2009), but their influence on the Indian tradition is not very evident. The underlying theme for genesis of illness in Ayurveda (Indian medicine) is similar to the humoral theories that underpinned thinking about madness and mental illness in Greek culture. In China too, a medical dimension to madness was recognized for centuries, although during the Qing Dynasty (1644–1911) the illness approach to madness was played down when the rulers decreed that madness should be treated as deviance (Ng, 1990). However, it is important to note that in Indian, Chinese and Islamic medicine, illness was always seen holistically. So, from the point of view of the people who were treated as 'ill', the meaning of illness vis-à-vis the person suffering it was crucial, whether the illness and the person suffering it were integral or separate: If illness and the person suffering it were integral, any spiritual and/or supernatural elements to causation, extraneous stresses, imbalance or disturbance of the humours and so on, all were part and parcel of the person who suffered illness, not separate elements or separate factors in aetiology.

Cause of ill-health

In a western tradition, the cause of mental illness is ultimately inside the psyche (or brain) or else in the environment; if it is the latter case, the effect on mental health would be determined by the action (of environment) on the psyche. This inside–outside division may not mean much in a holistic tradition where the two are interposed within each other, in which case what happens out there is felt as within oneself. Viewed from a traditional western outlook, the attribution of ill-health to (say) the behaviour of a stranger, movement of the stars or a natural event such as a clap of thunder, may be seen as a 'projection' of psychological problems on to the environment. But in a holistic way of thinking, causes of illness that are external may coexist with causes that are within the person who is ill. Considerable problems could arise in a multicultural setting, where alternative traditions exist side by side, in the course of discussion about causation (of illness) or during educational programmes.

Explanatory models

'Explanatory model' is a term coined by Kleinman (1980) to mean the (culturally normal) explanations for causation of illness. Boundaries between health and disease, and between mind and body, are drawn in different ways in different cultural traditions. As a result, the major causes of 'mental illness' (in western terms) may appear to be somato-psychic when classical Ayurvedic theories of Indian medicine are viewed from a western standpoint (Obeyesekere, 1977); and, similarly, some forms of human distress that are conceptualized in the West as 'illness' may be seen in religious or philosophical terms in the Indian tradition. In Tibetan thinking, based on the northern (Mahāyāna) Buddhist tradition, the most crucial psychological factor involved with insanity is the same as that required for pursuing enlightenment (Clifford, 1984): 'It all depends on whether or not it is accepted and comprehended and ultimately worked with as the key to liberation. If it is not, it becomes, because the realization is still there unconsciously, the cause of denial, repression and, ultimately, mental illness' (pp. 138–9). Although the western model of illness has developed in a Christian culture, it has no place for Christian concepts such as 'salvation' or 'damnation', because, in the West, religion and illness are in separate cultural compartments. This secular approach to illness is not seen in non-western cultural traditions. The overall worldview within a culture, appertaining to health, religion, psychology and spiritual concerns, determines the meaning within that culture of madness, mental illness and mental health. In African and Eastern traditions, and possibly in all non-western traditions, a spiritual dimension of human experience plays a large part in the rubric that encapsulates mental health, because religion and health are not separated as they are in western psychology.

The differences in cultural traditions outlined in this chapter are only a start. Each overarching 'culture' includes many variations and there are many cultures that may not even be addressed within the Asian–African–European trio; the panoply of cultures on the American continent and those indigenous to Australia are some.

Conclusions

Generalizing about cultural traditions is difficult and fraught. Cultures are never static; they get modified and undergo changes which are sometimes abrupt, especially in parts of the world that have been invaded and/or colonized recurrently. But a few basic tendencies can be abstracted: Writing for a western audience, Graham (1986) states, 'Eastern culture and its institutions are traditionally humanistic in the sense that they are centred around the human potential for transcendence or becoming' (p. 11). But eastern culture is not humanistic in the sense of idealizing the human being as an all-powerful individual, the sort of thinking that forms the (individualistic) basis of western culture. Religion and psychology are integrated in the traditional philosophies of Hinduism, Buddhism, Zen, Taoism and Islam. In the eastern tradition, rationality is seen as *maya*—illusory and superficial. Chinese philosophy sees reality, whose ultimate essence is called *tao*, as a process of continual flow and change. I believe such fundamentals of culture often persist in some form or other and also get transported when people move around, persisting in cultural diasporas around the world.

Although considering cultural differences is important for a book such as this one, it is important not to jump to conclusions about a person— or a 'cultural group' in terms of their 'culture'. Although, west/non-west differences are useful to keep in mind when planning services or treatments, danger arises when the individual is lost sight of in the search for their 'culture' or (something even more common) when cultural difference is assumed just by the way someone looks or speaks or behaves and cultural difference is presumed from apparent racial difference.

3
Medicalization of Human Problems in the West

According to historian Edward Shorter (1997): 'Before the end of the eighteenth century, there was no such thing as psychiatry' (p. 1), meaning that doctors who cared for inmates of institutions to house people deemed to be 'insane' (which had existed in Europe from the middle ages) did not work to a medical system as such but were purely custodians. But, Shorter ignores the medieval *māristāns* (Islamic hospitals) of North Africa and Spain referred to in Chapter 2, where organized medical treatment in the (Greek) Galenic tradition that was incorporated into Islamic medicine was provided for the patients, who were diagnosed mostly as suffering from melancholia (Dols, 1992). Also, Shorter seems to discount the work of Pinel in France in the 1790s, where asylum inmates were given psychological treatment (see below). Unfortunately, with the break-up of the Islamic empire and the consequent deterioration of the *māristāns*, anything resembling an Islamic medical system (for insanity as an illness) seemed to have disappeared, except for bits that survive in the *unani* tradition of India and western Asia ('the near-east' of Europeans); and the work of Pinel lost its impact in the French asylums as the gains of the French revolution dissipated.

In this chapter, I trace the process by which human problems became medicalized in western culture, the institutional structures that enabled this to happen and the creation of the medical discipline of psychiatry. After considering the scene in Europe and North America, I include a section on the racist tradition of psychiatry that still resonates in both Europe and North America and has implications for what is happening in the ex-colonial countries of Asia and Africa (Chapter 7). Finally, I trace the path (in Europe and North America) to current bio-medical psychiatry before drawing some conclusions. It should be noted that many people seen as 'insane' in Europe and the USA of the seventeenth and eighteenth centuries may not be seen today, in the twenty-first, as suffering from a mental illness as such. However, others—many more possibly because the scope of 'mental illness'/psychiatric disorder has broadened tremendously over the years—who were then seen as mentally healthy/free of any disorder as such may well today qualify for receiving one or other psychiatric diagnosis if they live in a place that is accessed by psychiatrists (people trained in western allopathic system of medicine that includes psychiatry) or within the scope of mental health services based on psychiatry.

Europe

It is true that many of the 'treatments' in medieval European asylums cannot be called 'medical', because they were not administered as remedies for illness as such but mainly for control and (probably) punishment. However, humanitarian zeal for social reform after the French revolution resulted in something very different (Davidson *et al.*, 2010). Philippe Pinel, a French physician best known for removing the chains of lunatics confined at the Salpêtrière Asylum (depicted in a painting by Fleury), was appointed as a doctor to the asylum at Bicêtre in the early 1790s. Pinel devised a therapeutic approach called *traitement moral* for the management of inmates of the asylum. *Traitement moral* is best translated into English as 'psychological therapy' since the French word *moral* was at that time closer to the English 'psychological' than 'moral' (Davidson *et al.*, 2010). Pinel formulated madness as something that arose from 'vivid sensitivity and from psychological qualities that we value highly' (Weiner, 1992, p. 728) and, together with Jean-Baptiste Pussin, an ex-patient and manager of the asylum, aimed to treat the inmates humanely with compassion and understanding. Pinel's (1806) *Treatise on Insanity* was an extraordinary document for its time not only for this very reason and for seeing madness as something quite natural, an understandable form of illness, but also for seeing people diagnosed with madness as very special people who needed protection from society until they got over their affliction sooner or later. However, the approach towards the insane that Pinel advocated did not last very long, if indeed it even spread very far from Paris itself. But some of these ideas, especially the humane approach to asylum inmates, crossed the English Channel to England, although 'moral treatment' that accompanied a humane approach—introduced at the asylum run by Quakers called The Retreat at York (Tuke, 1813)—was very different to Pinel's *traitement moral*, being essentially an educational approach whereby patients were trained in the 'morality' of the times. Pinel's revolutionary movement in Paris was soon submerged in a central European influence that evolved 'a comprehensive program of institutional therapy [range of individual therapies that could only be provided in institutions] ... that made psychiatry into a therapeutic profession' (Shorter, 1997, p. 14).

As asylums for lunatics grew in number in the nineteenth century (Chapter 2), they came under medical jurisdiction, and consequently some thought was given to identifying the forms of madness as different illnesses and thence devising forms of treatment and management of the illnesses, that is, a proper medical approach. The illnesses were seen as biologically derived and treatments were mainly physical in what came to be known as the German (later German-British) system of psychiatry of the nineteenth century. The medical doctors in charge of asylums, initially called 'alienists' in mainland Europe and 'mad doctors' in England (Bynum, 1981), were gradually recognized as (medical) psychiatrists and formed their own associations. In Britain, the Association of Medical Officers of Asylums, formed in 1841, changed its name to the Royal Medico-Psychological Association and finally became the Royal College of Psychiatrists in 1971. However, about the same time (late nineteenth and early twentieth centuries), Freudian psychoanalysis arrived on the scene promoting 'the notion that psychological problems arose as a result of unconscious conflicts over long-past events'; and 'for several decades, [some] psychiatrists were glad to adopt this theory of illness causation ... especially because it permitted them to shift the locus of psychiatry from the asylum to private practice' (Shorter, 1997, p. 145). Until recently, the 'talking therapies' that emanated from psychological theories of illness-causation was applicable only to people categorized as suffering 'neuroses'; and the 'psychoses' were largely left to hospital psychiatrists.

North America

With the destruction of the pre-Columbian cultures and the exclusion from mainstream society of what remained of the original inhabitants (who are sometimes called 'Indians' or Aborigines but will be referred to in this book as the First Nations of America or just 'First Nations'), North America became culturally, and in terms of the heritage of most of its people, an extension of Europe. The medical doctors of the First Nations were the shamans and they clearly had sophisticated knowledge of herbal remedies for disease and complex healing practices for (what today would be seen as) mental disorder (Gamwell and Tomes,

1995). But ideas about mental health among the First Nations were not allowed to influence practical service provision for mental health problems, even when the clients were people from the nations who wanted to maintain their own traditional ways. And European ideas about mental illness were forcibly imposed; for instance, homosexuality (which was accepted as 'normal' among people of most First Nations) 'was considered a crime in the seventeen and eighteenth centuries, and in the nineteenth century gradually came to be viewed as mental illness', and First Nations' doctors (shamans) were vilified as *berdashes*, the French word for male prostitutes (Gamwell and Tomes, 1995, p. 15). From the early days of Europeanization of the Americas, Africans were brought over as slaves. Their varied African traditions towards (what are now called) mental problems included the use of herbal remedies and religious healing, but all this knowledge was mostly lost although it survived for a time sporadically in slave communities (Gamwell and Tomes, 1995). The so-called melting pot of America was a graveyard of First Nations' cultures and the knowledge held in them; and for African-Americans and their cultural traditions, the results were equally tragic in a different way.

Early European colonists in the USA attributed (what is now seen as) mental illness to demonic possession and practised severe punishments for those afflicted. But as ideas from the (European) Enlightenment (see Chapter 2) came across the Atlantic, the medico-diagnostic approach to problems of living and individual behaviour became the cultural norm, exemplified by the first major American medical treatise on mental illness—*Medical Inquiries and Observations upon the Disease of the Mind*, first published in 1812 (Rush, 1818). European trends for establishing asylums (later called mental hospitals) followed; as in Europe these institutions initially provided custodial care only, but later various physical treatments were imported from Europe. However, an American counterpart to The Retreat at York was established in 1817 at Frankford Pennsylvania and called Friends Asylum; and the humane approach to lunatics first proposed by Pinel (see section 'Europe') was introduced in therapeutic houses that replaced asylums in some parts of the USA (Davidson *et al.*, 2010). As in the UK, psychiatrists banded together in an association which became the American Psychiatric Association in 1921. But, while in the UK and mainland Europe the dominant approach to psychiatry was bio-medical following the lead of Kraepelin (see section 'Lead-up to bio-medical psychiatry'), psychoanalytic ideas derived from Freud played a greater role in American psychiatry until recently (Chapter 6).

Racist tradition of psychiatry

Psychiatry developed at a time when white-on-black slavery was prevalent in most of South America, the southern states of the USA, the Cape regions of South Africa and the Caribbean. And ideas of 'race' interacted with practice of psychiatry to produce ways of thinking that fed into mainstream psychiatry itself. During times of slavery in the USA, an American physician Samuel Cartwright (1851) claimed that nearly all 'free negroes' were afflicted by a particular psychiatric disorder called *dysaesthesia aethiopis*: '[I]f they had not got some white person to direct and take care of them'—a disease apparently characterized by 'insensibility' of the skin and 'hebetude' of mind so that 'they break, waste, and destroy everything they handle ... raise disturbances with their overseers and fellow servants without cause or motive, and seem to be insensible to pain when subject to punishment' (p. 321). Another disease described by Cartwright was more straightforward—'Drapetomania or the disease causing slaves to run away' (p. 318). Almost into the twentieth century, Babcock (1895), a psychiatrist from South Carolina, while claiming that mental disease was 'almost unknown among savage tribes of Africa', attributed the alleged 'increase of insanity [among African Americans] since emancipation' to the deleterious effect of freedom on 'sluggish and uncultivated brains' and forecast 'a constant accumulation of [black] lunatics' in the years to come (pp. 423–7). Dr Arrah B. Evarts (1913), a physician at the Government Hospital for the Insane in Washington DC, wrote that the high levels of mental illness among African-Americans was a result of their being unable to cope with emancipation from slavery since Africans were 'child-like savages' (p. 393), a view that was typical of American opinion in the early twentieth century.

But racist thinking in psychiatry did not emanate from slavery alone. It was a common practice in psychiatric literature to designate anyone who was not of 'European stock' ('white race') as uncivilized; for example, Daniel Tuke (1858), renowned English psychiatrist who was a lecturer on psychological medicine at York and a medical officer to The Retreat at York, commented on what he called 'the statistics of insanity in uncivilized countries' (p. 105), meaning those in Africa and Asia. In his classic *Totem and Taboo*, Freud (1913) saw similarities between 'the mental lives of savages and [European] neurotics' (p. 276); and Devereux (1939), an anthropologist, viewed non-western healers (generally referred to as 'shamans') as neurotics or psychotics. Three distinct views about mental illness among non-Europeans were evident in the mid-eighteenth century: First, Daniel Tuke (1858) and Maudsley (1867, 1879) in England, Esquirol (cited by Jarvis, 1852) in France and Rush (cited by Rosen, 1968) in the USA voiced views reiterating Rousseau's concept of the 'noble savage'—that 'savages' who lacked the civilizing influence of western culture were free of mental disorder. Second, a stance evident in Europe was that non-Europeans were mentally degenerate because they lacked western culture (Lewis, 1965). Finally, epidemiological studies based on the Sixth US Census of 1840 (Anon, 1851) were used to justify a claim that the black person was relatively free of madness in a state of slavery but 'becomes prey to mental disturbance when he is set free' (Thomas and Sillen, 1972, p. 16). Although the 'noble savage' viewpoint idealized non-European culture in some ways and the 'degenerate primitive' attitude vilified it, both approaches sprang from the notion that European culture alone, associated with white races, was 'civilized'; the culture of black people, being 'primitive', rendered them either free of mental disorder or inherently degenerate. And then much later, European proponents of colonial psychiatry added to the racist psychiatric literature with comments around alleged underdevelopment of black and brown-skinned people (see Chapter 5).

Although not now stated overtly, the (racist) attribution of primitiveness to non-Europeans and to their cultures has persisted in the thinking of (western) psychiatry, being reflected in problems of institutional racism in psychiatric practice and research studies of the 1970s and 1980s (see Chapter 7). The assumption often made within psychiatry that western psychiatric concepts, illness-models and treatments have all got global relevance, seen, for example, in the so-called 'global' mental health approach (Chapter 8), subsumes within it an arrogance that reflects racist judgement about cultures and peoples (see Chapter 7).

Lead up to bio-medical psychiatry

The medical approach to madness (lunacy) that had developed in the Islamic Empire (Chapter 2) virtually disappeared by the mid- to late fifteenth century as that empire broke up. But medical study appertaining to mental illness emerged again in the late sixteenth century when the word *psychologia* began to be used in Europe (Zilborg, 1941) and medical interest in matters to do with the mind restarted again (as in Islamic medicine) around the idea of melancholia as an illness. In 1586, *A Treatise on Melancholy* by Timothy Bright appeared in England and, in 1621, *The Anatomy of Melancholy* by Robert Burton (1806). Medical psychology or psychological medicine, later called 'psychiatry', developed in European culture through two movements in thinking (Bynum, 1981): First, certain behavioural patterns and kinds of mental states were attributed to disease meriting medical interest, rather than to postulates such as possession by demons, a state of sin or wilful criminality; and second, there appeared the idea of the mind as an expression of brain activity. It was against this background that the asylum movement (Chapter 2) and 'the great confinement [of lunatics in asylums]' (Foucault, 1967, p. 38) took place. As the number of asylums grew in the seventeenth and eighteenth centuries, medical doctors in charge of them achieved a sort of constituency of people they controlled and, thus, a power base. They developed systems of diagnosis using whatever knowledge they could glean, including classical descriptions of illness by Hippocrates (Zilborg, 1941). Each asylum tended to develop its own classification, although the Congress of Mental Medicine in Antwerp in 1885 attempted to develop some uniformity by agreeing a list of categories that all those who attended the meeting agreed upon (Table 3.1) (Tuke, 1890). Basically, illnesses were constructed to explain groups of (what asylum doctors saw as) 'symptoms' in the people incarcerated in the asylums.

The main centre of academic study in Europe during the mid-nineteenth century was in Germany and, from 1883 onwards, Kraepelin produced systems of classification of mental illness based on observation of asylum patients. In the fifth edition of his textbook *Psychiatrie*, Kraepelin (1896) revived an idea about psychopathology initially put forward by Morel (1857) called 'degeneration' (see Chapter 2 for a discussion of this concept), to claim that an illness that he called 'dementia præcox' was the culmination of degeneration in an individual; and he

Table 3.1 Principal forms of madness agreed at Antwerp in 1889

Mania
Melancholia
Periodical insanity
Progressive systematic insanity
Dementia
Organic and senile dementia
General paralysis of the insane
Insane neurosis (hysteria, epilepsy, hypochondriasis and so on)
Toxic insanity
Moral and impulsive Insanity
Idiocy and similar conditions

Source: Based on Tuke (1890, p. 119).

divided this illness into different types called hebephrenia, catatonia, dementia paranoides and, in the eighth edition (Kraepelin, 1913), simple dementia, all caused by degeneration. In 1911, dementia præcox was renamed 'schizophrenia' by Bleuler (1950) as a subgroup of insanity which he reckoned resulted from a 'splitting of psychic functions' (1911, p. 9). Kraepelin is sometimes hailed as the 'father of modern [biological] psychiatry' (Weber and Engstrom, 1997, p. 1). The hallmark of his approach (sometimes called 'Kraepelian' or 'Kraepelinian') was the emphasis on genetic causes of mental illness and the search for physical treatments for insanity. The system of classification of mental illness led to two compendia of psychiatric nosology which are periodically updated, the current ones being the *ICD-10 Classification of Mental and Behavioural Disorders* (henceforth ICD-10) (WHO, 1992) and the *Diagnostic and Statistical Manual of Mental Disorders* (fifth edition, henceforth DSM-5) (APA, 2013). Psychiatric nosology in ICD-10 is summarized in Table 3.2, but DSM-5 is too complicated and extensive to be summarized in a simple table.

Although generally conforming to the traditional western approach to mental health and illness described in Chapter 2, the (psychiatric) profession, almost from the word go, and on both sides of the Atlantic, was split into hospital psychiatrists in charge of people given diagnoses such as psychosis, manic-depressive insanity and schizophrenia, and private psychiatrists, often having both hospital and private practices. However, from early days there were occasionally 'neurosis units' in asylums (especially those called mental hospitals). The predominant model for mental illness adopted on both sides of the Atlantic was the bio-medical one; but psychoanalytic influence played a greater role in the USA, whereas in

Table 3.2   ICD-10 classification of mental and behavioural disorders

Organic and symptomatic disorder
Mental and behavioural disorder due to substance abuse
Schizophrenia, schizotypal disorder and delusional disorder
Mood (affective) disorder
Neurotic, stress-related and somatoform disorder
Behavioural disorder associated with physiological disturbance
Disorder of adult personality and behaviour
Mental retardation
Disorder of psychological development
Behavioural and emotional disorder with childhood onset
Unspecified disorder

Source: Based on WHO (1992).

the UK the German (Kraepelian) influence dominated. However, some people diagnosed as suffering 'psychosis' were treated outside hospitals, especially if they were well-to-do or had rich or well-connected relatives. I worked in a couple of neurosis units under the National Health Service in and near London in the early 1960s. In my experience, the neurosis units catered for middle-class people and/or people who had consulted psychiatrists privately (paying fees) before being admitted to the neurosis unit; while people with very similar problems but unable to afford fee-paying psychiatry were housed in the general section of the hospital.

Hospital psychiatrists used various surgical and physical, sometimes electrical and chemical, methods for suppressing behaviour of patients that they (the psychiatrists) deemed unreasonable or disordered, believing that they were counteracting a biological processes causing illness. Most treatments were meant to shock the nervous system and/or control symptoms of illness such as delusions and hallucinations; but often it was not clear whether the treatment given within psychiatric settings was directed at symptoms or merely for control of behaviour, thought processes or beliefs. In fact, I think this confusion still prevails. This problem was evident in two of the most widely used (and, indeed, dramatic) procedures that have since then been abandoned, namely lobotomy (surgical severance of connections between two parts of the brain) and insulin coma therapy. In the former, people whose behaviour was seen as 'disturbed', that is, erratic and irrational, were converted by the operation into passive, easily managed people, but unfortunately often vegetable-like individuals. Insulin coma treatment (inducing hypoglycaemic comas with injections of insulin and then waking up comatose patients with intravenous glucose) was used for people diagnosed as suffering from schizophrenia (see Moncrieff, 1999) and probably caused brain damage (Whitaker, 2002). In fact, insulin coma treatment was not abandoned in the UK until the 1950s when a controlled trial found it to be no more effective than barbiturate-induced sleep (Ackner *et al.*, 1957), although I recall it being used extensively in Sri Lanka when I worked there in the early 1960s. ECT (electroconvulsive therapy), which is designed to initiate an epileptic fit, is still used although highly controversial (Moncrieff, 2009).

Throughout the first half of the twentieth century, a large number of 'mental patients' languished in state-run mental hospitals all over Europe often in poor conditions, frequently neglected and deprived of ordinary human rights, apparently impervious to 'treatment'; while, at the same time, psychoanalytic psychotherapy and other types of 'talking therapies' thrived in the private sector sometimes achieving (especially in North America) fashionable status. In the eyes of historian Shorter (1997), the 'physical therapies [for mental illness] represented a series of alternatives to the dilemma of custodialism versus psychoanalysis' but, 'for half a century [the first half of the twentieth] the discipline of psychiatry stood trapped between the choices of custodial care and individual psychoanalysis' (p. 238).

In the 1960s, it was noticed that psychiatric practice was rather different on the two sides of the Atlantic, especially in the way serious mental illness was diagnosed—a matter that was confirmed by the UK–US Diagnostic Project (Cooper *et al.*, 1972), using a standardized system of diagnostic interviewing called the Present State Examination devised by British psychiatrists (Wing *et al.*, 1974). As it became evident that drug treatment for schizophrenia was becoming popular, there was pressure to standardize the diagnostic system to achieve reliability of diagnoses across the Atlantic, and diagnoses based on specific definable symptoms was felt to be needed. This was the beginning of mainstream American psychiatry moving away from its psychoanalytic influences to fall into the European bio-medical tradition. Revision of DSM began to reflect this shift leading into the medication revolution in psychiatric treatment (Chapter 6).

Conclusions

The western notions of mental health and illness that emerged after the (European) Enlightenment fed into a medicalization of madness. The racism of post-Enlightenment Europe was reflected in a racist tradition in psychiatry reinforced during white-on-black slavery and then again during colonial times. During the twentieth century, especially its latter half, personal problems of living, thinking and behaving together with social and political issues that affected ordinary people resulted in the construction under the aegis of psychiatry of various personal 'illnesses' located in the mind. Psychiatry developed a little differently on the two sides of the Atlantic mainly because psychoanalysis was much more influential for quite some time in North America, whereas in most of Europe (except to some extent in France) the German-British school of bio-genetic psychiatry was dominant. However, the two came together soon after the end of the Second World War with moves towards standardizing the categorization of diagnostic practice (see Chapter 6).

Part II

What Happened in the Majority World

This part of the book describes the state of play in the non-western world until about the mid-twentieth century vis-à-vis the likely experience of people who may have had (in western psychiatric terms) mental health problems and mental illness. It examines what is known about the way problems and illnesses (seen in western cultural idioms as 'mental') may have been viewed in the non-western world and what help (or services) may have been available if needed. Also, it describes the impact of colonial psychiatry in terms of its effect on ordinary people and its legacy for the post-colonial era.

4
Mental Health and Mental Illness in Non-Western Countries

It is difficult to set mental health and ill-health (as understood today in the English-language literature and discourse) in a proper historical context worldwide because the language of mental health and illness has come about in a very limited part—primarily *European*—of a culturally diverse universe with its medical and psychological traditions being influenced very much by (western) *psychiatry* (see Chapters 2 and 3). In other words, the discourse in the field of mental health is articulated in the form of concepts mostly embedded in Euro-American psychiatry. The concepts around mind, illness and health in other cultures—those of the Majority World—that would approximate, or be similar to, 'mental health' and 'mental illness' (as understood in the language of psychiatry) are often very different (Chapter 2). As a result, it is not easy to fathom what exactly was going on in the past, nor indeed the present situation, vis-à-vis 'mental health' in non-western low- and middle-income countries (LMICs)/the Global South (see 'Introduction' for use of language), since, in these non-western cultures, what is seen as 'mental health' in Anglo-American English is often not articulated in the language of health and ill-health alone, but mostly in language applicable to social relationships, religion, ethics, philosophy/spirituality or just ordinary non-technical everyday terms. Epidemiological research using psychiatric models of illness—and most researchers use these—are of very limited value, some would say practically useless cross-culturally, mainly because of 'category fallacy' (Kleinman, 1977) and other problems in cross-cultural research outlined below. The literature in cultural anthropology on ritual healing is difficult to relate to 'mental health'; healing is mostly about generalized problems encountered by individuals that include 'illness' as well as other misfortunes from which the supplicant may want to be free of (liberated from) unlike the case of people who seek treatment for 'illness'. And in any case, healing in non-western settings is described (for western audiences) mainly by anthropologists and they (anthropologists) have little interest in outcomes, unlike psychiatrists and medical people who invariably look for outcomes from 'treatment' since 'outcome' is an important concept in the language of illness.

My intention in this chapter is to work out what it may have been like in the past for people in LMICs, for example, in Asia and Africa, who would (by today's psychiatric criteria) be diagnosed as suffering from mental illness or mental health problems. There is little or no evidence, anecdotal or otherwise, that we could garner from stories of people in Asian and African countries in pre-colonial times who may have suffered 'mental illness' (as described in psychiatry) because the constructions that form (western) 'mental illness' did not exist in non-western cultures. So, what I do in this chapter is to make some informed guesses, based on reviewing information we have of living standards, cultures and social conditions of people in Asian and African regions which now comprise LMICs, focusing on the point of this exercise which is to draw some conclusions about those who may have required help with equivalents of (in today's terminology) 'mental problems' or 'mental illness', whatever these may have been called in other places at other times.

As a start, I discuss the making of what came to be called the 'Third World', that graduated into being called 'developing countries' and then LMICs (see 'Introduction' for discussion of points about language). For this discussion, I shall refer to recent revisionist literature rather than repeating traditional misconceptions about the 'non-West' that are often passed off as historical facts. Then, I present critically some cross-cultural international studies that enable us to understand the differences and similarities that exist in this field; and after that I consider some of the evidence about healing that relate to (what we now call) 'mental health'. I follow this with a section on various bits of evidence appertaining to the main issues being pursued in this chapter and a section outlining what was likely to have been available in the way of medical treatment in the pre-colonial Third World Finally, I draw some conclusions on what life was probably like vis-à-vis mental health and illness (as we know these topics in western terminology) for people living in the Global South in pre-colonial and medieval times in the light of the evidence from the information covered and the reality of cultural diversity in understandings of mental health and illness.

The Third World and its underdevelopment

Although the term 'underdevelopment' should be limited to industrialization or economic status, it tends to slip into being given wider, often pejorative, meaning denoting social and cultural states. So 'underdeveloped' countries are sometimes assumed to be 'primitive' with underdeveloped social systems and even cultures, connecting with racist ideas about peoples and nations that reflect misconceptions strongly held well into the late twentieth century and fairly prevalent even in the twenty-first. The question for us is about standards of living and quality of life for people in Asia and Africa before they were colonized by western powers in the late seventeenth century.

A view widely held in the West but shown to be largely mistaken is that countries of Asia, Africa and South America have *always* been 'underdeveloped' until modern post-colonial times; even Karl Marx (1978) wrote in 1853 that India's 'social condition has remained unaltered since its remotest antiquity until its final decennium of the 19th century [of British colonization]' (p. 656). Fortunately, several writers have placed new books in the public domain outlining the true picture of economic conditions in what became European colonies. There is hardly any need to point out that Indian and Chinese societies were highly sophisticated (for the times) both socially and culturally during the middle-ages when Europe was relatively backward, but what is often not realized is that the Islamic Empire of North Africa and Southern Spain achieved a high standard of cultural development too at that time—see, for instance, *The Islamic Middle East* by Charles Lindholm (1996).

Living standards in East and West

Kenneth Pomeranz (2001) shows that, as recently as 1750, Asia, compared to Europe, had a higher life expectancy and consumption of consumer goods. In other words, Asian people in the sixteenth and seventeenth centuries enjoyed better standards of living (Bairoch, 1981) than Europeans did. At 1700, China, India and Europe had about equal share (roughly 23 per cent) of world Gross Domestic Product (GDP) according to Angus Maddison (1998). Economically, India was relatively well off with exports of high quality consumer goods to Europe: Parthasarathi (2011) points out that the banking system, set up by the Mughal Empire of sixteenth and seventeenth centuries that covered most of India except the South (Berinstain,1998), enabled easy access to capital—as the (British) East India Company found in the nineteenth century. The caste system which came to stifle social and commercial progress later on was neither rigid nor very prominent in the seventeenth and eighteenth centuries; its rigidity occurred with the 'colonial transformation of Indian society' (Parthasarathi, 2011, p. 59).

Like India, China too was relatively prosperous in the 200 years before incursions of the European powers. Mike Davis (2001) quotes Pomeranz as providing evidence that eighteenth century Chinese enjoyed higher standards for consumption and lower mortality rates when compared to Europeans of the time. Unlike India, where the economy deteriorated as colonization began to bite with breakup of the Mughal Empire in the eighteenth century, Chinese GDP grew much faster than its European counterpart throughout the eighteenth century and its share of world GDP in 1820 was *higher* than that of Europe (Maddison, 1998). The downward trend in the Chinese economy began in the aftermath of the mid-nineteenth century 'opium wars', imposed on China by western powers in order to force easy imports into China of opium from British India so that Chinese consumer goods could be purchased for Europe. This was called 'free trade' (Jacques, 2012, p. 48). According to Davis (2001), in 1868

> the chain worked like this: The United Kingdom paid the United States for cotton by bills upon the Bank of England. The Americans took some of these bills to Canton and swapped them for tea. The Chinese exchanged the bills for [British-]Indian opium. Some of the bills were remitted to England as profit; others were taken to India to buy additional commodities, as well as to furnish the money remittance of private fortunes in India and funds for carrying on the Indian government at home. (p. 300)

The main manufacturing districts in the world up to the time of colonialism were in the Yangsi Delta (China), and in India, Bengal, Gujarat and Madras (now called Chennai) District were not far behind (Parthasarathi, 2011; Pomeranz, 2001): 'India alone produced one-quarter of world manufactures'; and Indian commercial capital in some ways surpassed even that of China (Davis, 2001, p. 292). Trade was a one-way affair: 'In the world economy of the seventeenth and eighteenth centuries, silver flowed from west to east, balanced by the opposite flow of manufactured goods. And from the seventeenth century Europeans faced sustained competition from Asian imports, including cotton textiles, porcelains, ships, silks and even fans and furniture' (Parthasarathi, 2011, p. 10). That was of course before colonization changed the balance.

The underdevelopment of Asia leading eventually to its current relative poverty started with colonization; in other words economic development, starting from a higher level anyway compared to the West, would almost certainly have proceeded at a normal pace during the eighteenth, nineteenth and twentieth centuries, if not for changes imposed after colonization. While Asian colonies were underdeveloped, the white settler colonies of Australia, Canada and New Zealand were 'always treated entirely differently—for straightforward racial and eth-nic reasons—and prospered greatly as a consequence' (Jacques, 2012, p. 49). However, some changes during colonization set the stage for post-colonial economic development. For example, India obtained a widely shared language of English and China gained some knowledge of European commerce from the treaty ports such as Shanghai. And, of course the British colonial government developed the Indian Railways and China eventually benefited from the international trading centre called Hong Kong.

The story of Africa and South America

The underdevelopment of Africa is a somewhat different story. In his ground-breaking book *How Europe Underdeveloped Africa*, Walter Rodney (1988) traces the variety of sub-Saharan African cultures in the 500 years before European colonization in the late nineteenth century. Soci-eties were predominantly agricultural and even the riches of the great empires of Africa depended on agriculture and, latterly, gold mining. The widespread system of communalism in land ownership (similar to that in Asia) meant that 'every African was assured of sufficient land to meet his own needs by virtue of being a member of a family or community'; this meant that there were 'few social pressures or incen-tives for technical changes to increase productivity' and, unlike in Asia and North Africa, 'even the most politically developed [sub-Saharan] African states did not play the role of initiators and supervisor of agricul-tural development' (1988, p. 41). Manufacturing remained small-scale and of high quality; 'local cottons from the Guinea coast were [rep-utably] stronger than Manchester cottons' and cloth made from bark and palm fibre in the old kingdom of Kongo were said to have 'a finish comparable to velvet' (p. 42). In medieval times, lines of trade criss-crossed the Sahara and West Africa, connecting with the caravan routes from Middle-East that came from India and China (Davidson, 1984). European piracy along the West African coast in early fifteenth century was associated with trade in ivory, gold, pepper, and other goods but soon, the Portuguese, and later other Europeans, started looking for slaves.

Finally we come to the African holocaust that followed on the discovery of the American continent by Europeans. The need for cheap labour led to slavery organized by mainly British merchants aided by local African collaborators in what became the Atlantic slave trade (Davidson, 1984). In fact, the slave trade was probably a major factor in both African underdevelopment and European development. Between 1445 and 1870, about ten million Africans landed alive in America but the death rate in the 'middle-passage' (across the Atlantic) averaged 10 to 20 per cent and also many Africans captured by slavers died during captivity before transportation (Rodney, 1988; Walvin, 1992). The loss to the African labour force and the destruction and sorrow inflicted on African families and societies was only matched in an opposite direction by the massive wealth accumulated by European nations, the building of stable families with vast wealth and country mansions among the middle-classes in places like England, and the capital to finance the industrial revolution and ship-building that enabled the plunder that followed of Asia and (again) Africa during colonization.

The situation in South America, another part of the non-western world that suffered from western onslaught, is very different historically to both Africa and Asia. The Spanish conquests to destroy the highly developed empires of the region in order to extract wealth (taken back to Spain) did not finance industrialization but enabled the Christian empires to subdue (and drive out of Europe) Jews and Moslems and eventually decimate the Islamic cultures of North Africa, where, incidentally, the first organized medical approaches to 'madness' began (Chapter 2). As a result of the racial and cultural mixing that has taken place since Columbus landed in (what was to Europe) the 'new world', South America, as an unique multicultural and multiracial mix of people, has developed a cultural and political identity that separates it from Europe and North America, identifying it as a part of the Third World. Meanwhile, North America, rich and prosperous, closely tied up economically, culturally and politically with Western Europe now forms the dominant part of a Euro-American bloc, where biomedical approaches to mental health predominate (Chapters 2 and 3) and from where these are being exported to LMICs (Chapters 6, 7 and 8).

Problems of international research

Cross-cultural research in the field of mental health is fraught with practical problems. The main issue (especially for people using traditional quantitative research methods) is around 'category fallacy', a term coined by Arthur Kleinman (1977) to designate the error in taking a category of (mental) illness that may have some use in one cultural and social setting (say the UK or the USA) and using it in a very different location and sociocultural context (say in Africa or Asia). The basic problem has been described simply by Carstairs and Kapur (1976):

> A psychiatric symptom may be simply defined as a mental state which is perceived as odd, distressful or harmful by the person suffering it, or by those around him [or her], or both. What is odd or distressful or harmful to members of one cultural group may not be so regarded by members of another one. (pp. 11–12)

The authors cited in this quotation, Morris Carstairs and Ravi Kapur, carried out a study in the early 1970s that tried to get round the problem of category fallacy, but did so only partially. This study was written up (by them) as *The Great Universe of Kota: Stress, Change and Mental Disorder in an Indian Village* (Carstairs and Kapur, 1976) and is described more fully in Chapter 7. The researchers began by establishing what the communities they were researching in considered and felt were symptoms of sickness that needed intervention; and then they investigated how people in the communities sought help with their problems. Category fallacy is perhaps still the most important issue in international and cross-cultural research in mental health; most researchers approach cross-cultural research top-down by imposing model of illness often in the form of diagnoses based on psychiatric categories and this approach can lead to very misleading conclusions. The result is that a great deal of what goes for 'research findings' in cross-cultural and international research in the field of mental health and illness has to be viewed with some scepticism.

Apart from category fallacy, there are other important issues that need addressing in cross-cultural research. Even if there is no obvious language barrier and so no need for interpreters, misunderstandings emanating from subtle differences in the use of words could easily influence significantly conclusions drawn in research. Further, a word or set of words used in one language to articulate a particular emotional state or problem may not be translatable accurately to another language because the concepts that underlie them are 'ethnocentric', that is specific to a particular culture and its historical antecedents. Thus, it is often said that what the western world understands by 'depression' emanates from its Judeo-Christian (cultural) past and it is acknowledged that the cross-cultural validity of depression as a diagnostic category has not been established outside western culture (Kleinman and Good, 1985b); using literal translations of western concept 'depression' into non-European languages do not do justice to either side. Also, there are many non-western constructs around emotions that just cannot be translated at all into English; and similarly there are concepts that get distorted and misused when translated carelessly from one language to another. I mean, for example, the anomalous situation that arises when the Buddhist concept of 'mindfulness'—a non-judgemental observation of thoughts experienced in the course of meditation—is isolated as a sort of psychological technology to be added on to a form of behaviour therapy to form 'mindfulness cognitive behaviour therapy' (MCBT) (Crane, 2009). The practice of mindfulness in Buddhism (see Gunaratne, 2002) is very different to what is incorporated into its translation (as it were) in MCBT that is marketed as a technique for restructuring thought processes (Fennel, 2009; Scott and Beck, 2008). It is not just a matter of a partial loss in translation but more a matter of misuse (or abuse) of words and concepts. In many cross-cultural situations, observer bias can be a major issue if the people who do the research, and/or analyse results, come from very different backgrounds to those of the subjects of research and, even more importantly, carry biases and pre-conceptions emanating from racial and/or cultural stereotyping.

Another issue that results in mistakes in cross-cultural research is the failure to take on board the fact that many people in LMICs approach various systems of help (including religious and traditional healing) once they decide to seek help for (what we call but they may well not call) mental health problems. For instance in South Asia, pluralism in help-seeking is the norm (Halliburton, 2004; Nichter, 1980; Sachs, 1989; Tribe, 2007; Waxler, 1984; Waxler-Morrison, 1988); Vogt (1999), a psychotherapist who studied indigenous healing in the Kandyan region (Central Province) of Sri Lanka lists several types of healing that focus on (what we call) mental health problems (Table 4.1). Clearly the mix would be different in other places and in many Asian settings, such a list would include Western and Ayurvedic systems of medicine, astrological consultation, healing rituals, religious rituals and advice from religious counselors and so on. Differences in help-seeking practices coupled with

Table 4.1   Healing systems in the Kandyan region of Sri Lanka

Western (allopathic) medicine
Ayurvedic medicine
Healing rituals such as *Thovil, pujas*
Astrological consultation, fortune-telling, spirit-healing,
   instruction to perform rituals
Practical advice based on (Buddhist) *dhamma*
Pirit rituals, meditation (including mindfulness)

Source: Adapted from Vogt (1999, p. 12).

variations in types of service available could easily affect international studies of all types. Incorrect deductions may be made when researching a question about outcomes and benefit derived from 'treatment' because these concepts may be understood very differently in non-western cultural settings; traditional healers fulfil many functions in a society and do not merely deal with 'illness', which too is subsumed within a general category of 'misfortune'. The complexity of researching such situations is illustrated by the in-depth study of patient by anthropologist Amarasingham (1980)—a story too long to relate here but well worth reading up.

A well-known study carried out by the World Health Organization (WHO) in the 1970s is worth mentioning although category fallacy was ignored in its implementation—the International Pilot Study of Schizophrenia (IPSS) (WHO, 1973, 1975, 1979), described in more detail in Chapter 7. The aim of WHO at the time was to obtain information on how 'schizophrenia' (assumed incorrectly at the time to be a valid universal concept of illness) manifested in various regions of the world and what happened in terms of outcomes of people allegedly affected by the illness. (The organizers of the project did not question the validity of using the 'schizophrenia' diagnosis to identify psychiatric illness, a clear instance of category fallacy.) What WHO discovered was that people diagnosed with schizophrenia had a better outcome (judged on the basis of 'improvement' in symptoms) in non-western developing countries, when compared to those in relatively rich western countries. Views on cross-cultural research have changed somewhat since that study was carried out. It is now realized that 'culture' itself is not a fixed entity but subject to continuous change. This means that cultural changes need to be taken on board in both planning research and analysing results; and that cultural change interacts with psychological need and need for help at an individual level. Also, it is evident that aetiological models underlying mental distress and the manner in which social stresses may affect people may vary cross-culturally. For example, people in some cultural settings experience psychological trauma *collectively*, rather than as individual distress alone (Somasundaram, 2007) and community interventions (rather than individual 'treatment') may be required to deal with that (Fernando and Weerackody, 2009). (The difference between 'collective trauma' and 'individual trauma' is discussed in Chapter 10.)

Studies of healing

In most non-western traditions, there is interplay and overlap between medical and religious healing. There are extensive descriptions and analyses of religious healing in anthropological literature for example by Hobart (2003), Kapferer (1991) and Sax (2009). It is beyond the scope of this chapter to draw out general themes in healing across the world except to say that healing is closely connected with other aspects of culture in which a particular system (of healing) is embedded. Therefore, it is quite unrealistic to think of extracting a healing system from one cultural location and introducing it into another. Knowledge of healing indigenous to a particular place must form part of the background local knowledge that is required when mental health systems are being developed. For this, there needs to be connection between anthropological research and mental health research plus of course input from local people. (The importance of local knowledge when planning mental health services is discussed in Chapter 10.)

Tibet, as a landlocked and geographically isolated place, developed a system of medicine that was (and is) unique, different to both Indian and Chinese medical systems, although drawing from both. The system of healing for madness within Tibetan Medicine has been dubbed 'Tibetan Psychiatry' by Clifford (1984). She calls it a 'psychiatry' because teachings of orthodox Buddhism, or rather the elaboration of these in Tibetan Buddhism, were combined with herbal therapy and diet, derived from Ayurveda (one of the main Indian systems of medicine), to form a system of person-centred treatment for mental and emotional problems, including madness: 'A complex interweaving of religion, mysticism, psychology, and rational medicine' (p. 7). As in Ayurveda, aetiology was grounded in humoral theory (disease being seen as a reflection of humoral imbalance) but 'mental defilements', such as ignorance, unawareness, aversion and craving, were seen as causing changes in humoral balance. This relationship between the humours and human shortcomings as understood in Buddhist teaching, was indicative of the basic theory of psychosomatic relationships in the Tibetan system. Different treatments and medicines were applied to influence the mind through the body while (Buddhist) Dharma was not only the basis for judging mental functioning but also the basis for maintaining mental health.

A patient seeking help from a Tibetan medical practitioner would have been assessed for their humoral type (constitution) as well as the causes of the illness for the specific individual; and causes sought were not of the illness *per se* but of the illness in the individual. In Tibetan medicine, causes of illness may be ignorance, poisoning of the mind, unhealthy diet, environmental changes or a mixture of some or all of these (Rinpoche and Kunzang, 1973). According to Clifford (1984), the Tibetan doctor would look for a pattern of living 'that runs counter to one's [the patient's] inherent disposition' (p. 137); and the client and their relatives would receive advice on diet and (Buddhist) Dharma. But for more serious problems (of perhaps 'possession'), Tibetan psychiatry has a complex system of classification of demons that cause (what were seen as) illness equivalents to different types of psychoses (in western psychiatry): 'To the Tibetans, "demon" is a symbolic term. It represents a wide range of forces and emotions which are normally beyond conscious control and all of which prevent well-being and spiritual development' (p. 148). All the special tantric procedures for expelling demons (ritualized in exorcism) were in essence different expressions of compassion and emptiness—hence the importance of Dharma in developing the former and dealing with the latter). Clifford uses psychoanalytic images to see psychosis from a Tibetan medical perspective: Problems could build up into 'a tremendous panic... [associated with]... repression that is elaborated in terms of ego and unconscious tendencies... eventually leading to psychosis' (p. 138). Clifford goes on:

> Herein lies the crucial point. The psychological basis of insanity is the same basis for enlightenment. It all depends on whether or not it is accepted and comprehended and ultimately worked with as the key to liberation. If it is not, it becomes, because the realization is still there subconsciously, the cause of denial, repression and, ultimately, mental illness. (pp. 138–9)

It strikes me that people who accessed this sort of healer would have received a unique form of psychotherapy (for what a western-trained psychiatrist would call psychosis); but of course we do not know how easy it was for people in Tibet to get this treatment.

It was noted by Anthropologist Patricia Lawrence (2003) that in the face of deaths and disappearances in Sri Lankan Eastern coastal villages during the conflict (civil war) there that ended in 2009, attendance at Hindu temples to seek the help of the goddess Kali was a means of treatment for (what psychiatrists may call) 'depression' arising from grief and loss; and also a means by which bereaved people and women seeking their missing relatives found (what to them would be) treatment for their misfortune. The help they received was through oracular utterances of women who had been possessed by the goddess, and some indication of where they (the disappeared) may be. Lawrence's anthropological-psychological interpretation of good outcomes (that people who sought help had benefitted in lived experience) was that 'oracular revelations is a cultural confluence where many possibilities meet—where suffering and death are acknowledged, where courage can be instilled, where information about the future and protection might be given' (p. 119). This type of help-seeking and help-receiving has clearly been going on for a very long time. There is no reason to think that the type of 'treatment' described by Lawrence is any less effective today than it might have been in the past.

Even today in many Asian settings there are places of religious worship in various faiths that are well-known for healing people with mental illness. It is very likely that such places were much easier to access (and probably more numerous) in pre-colonial days than they are now. But current evidence collected from a psychiatric point of view may be more convincing than personal recollections collected by anthropologists, so I quote in the next paragraph just two studies that I know of. It should be noted that barriers to getting this sort of research funded and the difficulties of getting reports like this published in reputable English-language journals means that what could be 'evidence' of non-western treatment modalities remains largely hidden.

In the early 2000s, a paper by Raguram *et al.* (2002) in the *British Medical Journal* described outcomes of people who had attended a Hindu temple in Tami Nadu (South India) known for helping people with mental health problems. The authors had elicited the views of both the patients and their carers about their experiences and also made psychiatric assessments (of the patients) on a standard psychiatric scale before and after their stay at the temple. They found that most of the patients studied (a) suffered from psychotic illness (diagnosed by psychiatric methods) and (b) showed a degree of improvement (judged by reduction of psychiatric symptoms and their own expressed views) that matched the sort of result that may be expected by bio-medical therapy.

A couple of years later, a paper by Halliburton (2004) in the journal *Transcultural Psychiatry* documented the experiences of 100 people who had accessed treatment in three forms of therapy in Kerala (South India), namely Ayurvedic medicine, bio-medical psychiatry and religious healing at one or other of three locations, namely a Hindu temple, a Muslim mosque and a Christian church, all of which had reputations for healing people who suffer from mental illness. All the people who sought help had mixtures of symptoms that amounted to the diagnosis 'schizophrenia' or other severe mental disorder. Similar proportions of patients benefitted from each form of therapy, and several had changed from one to another until they derived benefit. This shopping around had resulted in a very high overall improvement rate.

Anecdotal/incidental evidence

We have glimpses about 'mental health' in Asian settings in the past by studying texts on Ayurveda (the main system of medicine on the Indian subcontinent), first written up 5,000 years ago (Jaggi, 1981; Sharma and Dash, 1983, 1985; Valiathan, 2003). Ayurveda refers to forms of madness as illness, but madness described in Ayurveda does not equate with 'madness' described in psychiatric literature. Very little is known for certain about African medicine in ancient times; but there, as well as in pre-Columbian America, advanced healing systems were probably available for people who required some intervention for (what is now called) 'mental illness', interventions described within the realms of religion as well as medicine (see Gelfand, 1964; Last and Chavunduka, 1986). In all these non-western settings of the ancient world, ideas and concepts about what today would be called 'mental illness' were represented in philosophy and religion as well as, to a limited extent, in indigenous medicine; and in any case, all illness was holistic, affecting all aspects of the person at the same time. In many instances there was little distinction between what (in modern terms) would be designated as misfortune, illness and spiritual crisis or experience. (The concept 'holism' is relation the health and illness is discussed in Chapter 2.) As far as I know, there were no 'mental hospitals' as such in India, China and the Americas before European influence; sickness of the 'mind' as something distinct from sickness of the body and problems of the spirit was not clearly recognized. However, mental hospitals did exist in the Islamic Empire of North Africa and Spain (see below and Chapters 2 and 3).

There is no evidence that people who may today be designated as 'mentally ill' (following psychiatric ways of classifying problems) in ancient Asian, African or American societies were dealt any less (or more) compassionately or effectively than they were in ancient European societies. Chapter 2 referred to some of the roots of the western system being in ancient Greece, and to mental hospitals (*māristāns*) of medieval Islamic Empire of the tenth to the thirteenth centuries. It is evident in reading the work of Dols (1992) that patients in the *māristāns* did not have the sorts of symptoms that western psychiatry identifies as hallmarks of (what it calls) severe mental illness—such as delusions and hallucinations.

According to Dols (1992) the *māristāns* in the Islamic empire were very different to European asylums built in Europe over 500 years later. They were impressive buildings with pools, fountains, flowing water and flower gardens. Unlike European asylums they were not isolated institutions but always in the centre of cities, easily accessible to most people. Clearly, the inmates ('patients') were frequently visited by family and friends and more generally seen as a part of society. As far as we know, these institutions were not used for confinement of people seen as socially undesirable as was the case with European asylums (see Chapters 2 and 3). The original *māristāns* building at Aleppo (in Syria) was reported as being used as a (western-type) mental hospital until recently (Maziak, 2006).

The conditions for residents ('patients') of the *māristāns* were apparently fairly good. It seems that great care was taken to decorate the wards to 'cheer the deranged'; there were 'beds with mattresses'; space for patients to wander about in; and reports of special food being supplied to patients at the Caliph's expense. However, there is no doubt that physical restraint was used on some people in the *māristāns*; visitors had sometimes reported observing beatings and there were reports of patients being held 'in iron chains until their reason is restored' (p. 119). Dispensing of medicines was common; stimulants, sedatives and drugs for 'gladdening of the spirit' being used (p. 133). Interestingly, it seems that music was used to treat melancholia, reflecting a medico-musical tradition (described in the Bible) going back to David treating Saul with music.

Coming to more recent times, the popular idea that nothing much was done about psychological or mental problems in pre-colonial Asia and Africa is probably untrue—as untrue I would think as the popular idea that people we would call 'mentally ill' were invariably persecuted in these societies in the way (say) witches were burned in medieval Europe. During most of the colonial period, indigenous medical therapies and even religious healing were actively suppressed by colonial governments in Asia, Africa and America, but some rudimentary mental hospitals (modelled on European asylums) were established in British and French colonies. Colonial psychiatry is covered in Chapter 5 but some snippets of information from that period are appropriate here.

In the 1950s, Margaret Field (1960), a doctor and anthropologist working for the British colonial office, described Ashanti shrines in Ghana where people with 'fear and guilt frenzies' and people who were (as she put it) 'indistinguishable from classical schizophrenics' benefitted from attending (p. 1045). I remember being told about a Buddhist temple at Neelammahara near Colombo, Sri Lanka, where a healer-priest practised Ayurvedic treatment for *unmada* (classical Ayurvedic equivalent to madness) (see Obeyesekere, 1977) using mainly herbal therapies combined with social care by local villagers boarding patients in their homes. Neelammahara Temple thrived as a centre for the healing of mental illness well into the 1980s. It is well known that there are today numerous centres in Asian and African countries where 'mad' people are taken for cures; this tradition of (religious) healing goes back a long way, the healing centres being usually around a temple, mosque or church. There is little doubt that people who are today designated as suffering 'insanity' or psychosis would then (in pre-colonial times and if they were thought to benefit from it) have been treated in one or other healing service, as indeed they are still in many LMICs, apparently often successfully, although we do not have definite evidence.

Pre-colonial Third World

The mental health scene (if we can call it that) in pre-colonial Third World would obviously have been very different to that in medieval Europe or present-day Europe, and indeed somewhat different to that in the Global South today. In order to be brief, I focus here on Asia and Africa, which after all forms the bulk of the Global South. We know something about the traditions that people there inherited (Chapter 2), and we know (earlier this chapter) what the regions were like in pre-colonial times in terms of living standards of people there. I suggest that we could fairly reliably draw a picture of what life may have been like vis-à-vis mental health and illness (as we know these topics today) for people in those regions during the 100 odd years before colonialism impacted on them. Clearly, people would have had various problems of living and some people would have been seen as 'mad'.

Different regions of the world (East and West, North and South) have influenced each other from time immemorial, but before colonialism and whatever globalization (see Chapter 1 for discussion of the term 'globalization') took place, the influence would have been mainly (what I call in Chapter 1) 'passive globalization', a sort of natural exchange of cultural forms and the permeation of ideologies across cultures. It is likely too that some of the problems seen as 'mental illness' in the West, including 'depression' of today and perhaps 'melancholia' of the past (see Chapter 2) were (and still are) normalized in some cultural settings by what Obeyesekere (1990) calls 'work of culture' (1990, title page). In the case of depression Obeyesekere (1985), an anthropologist, postulates the following explanation: He suggests that 'a painful series of affects pertaining to sorrow' may be universally identifiable in all societies; in the West, 'they are relatively free-floating... not anchored to an ideology and therefore identifiable and conducive to labelling as illness', while in some West African cultures and in the Sinhala-Buddhist culture (of Sri Lanka), these are 'intrinsically locked into larger cultural and philosophical issues of existence and problems of meaning' (p. 135) and therefore not 'illness', being dealt with naturally within the culture.

To judge by the evidence quoted in earlier paragraphs of this chapter, the pre-colonial world in Asia and Africa was highly developed (for their time) economically, socially and culturally. They were *civilized* places—using the word 'civilized' in the sense of being refined and enlightened—where human beings would have been valued and respected at least as much as, or possibly more than, they might have been in medieval Europe. For example, there is no evidence that the brutalities connected with how mental health was seen in medieval Europe, such as burning of witches or the inquisition of the Catholic Church, existed in (say) the Mughal Empire in India or the Empire of Mali in West Africa. Another difference between Europe and Asia/Africa of that period (in the sixteenth and seventeenth centuries, for instance) is that the latter had not experienced the so-called (European) 'Enlightenment' (discussed in Chapter 2) that resulted, among many other changes in ways of thought, in excluding religious traditions that valued spirituality, and strengthening individuality at the expense of communal feelings (Eze, 1997; Fernando, 2010; Morrison, 1993; Roger, 1994). It is safe to assume that anyone seen as requiring medical help in pre-colonial Asia and Africa would have received fairly high levels of care (for the time). Basham (1976) quotes evidence of medical establishments having been present in many parts of ancient and medieval Asia. South Indian inscriptions of the twelfth century AD refer to many medical centres for treatment of the sick, some with schools of medicine attached to them; there were over 100 hospitals in the Khmer kingdom, now Cambodia, in the twelfth century AD. Rulers such as the Indian Emperor Asoka (c.299 BC–c. 237) and the fourth-century Sri Lankan King Buddhadasa were particularly well known for their solicitude for the health of the populations they ruled over. Many of the medical establishments in India and Sri Lanka had been attached to temples and to some extent this tradition has continued to the present day. The trained physicians of ancient India were the *vaidyas*, 'a fraternity of men drawn from various classes and castes . . . . united by a common training and discipline for the high purpose of promoting human health and welfare' (Basham, 1976, p. 36). In ancient times the *vaidyas* were highly respected and of high status.

Societies in Asia and Africa, being predominantly family based and communal rather than individualistic (for discussion of individualism and collectivism, see Triandis, 1995), what are now seen as 'mental problems' (problems of the mind) would have been seen largely as being located 'out there', in the world around the individual, rather than inside their head or in the brain; largely ones of interaction with members of the family or community; not as personalized illness. And the spiritual dimension of human life being important, some problems of living and subjective feelings (for example, hearing voices) would have been attributed to supernatural forces, or at least causes outside human understanding, and not as breakdown in personal thinking processes; or else, they would have been interpreted in terms of emotional 'feel' for other people or connections with forces external to oneself. So the construction of problems of living as individualized mental illness (basically loss of reasoning) would have been minimal. In that sense, people who in the West were seen as 'mentally ill' requiring 'treatment' would have been facing (say) problems of living or existence. If they needed help, they would have turned to family or community or, if outsiders were required, there would have been various healing/consulting agencies. People seen as 'mad' may well have been looked after if they had family, but some may have been neglected or even excluded from society. If seen as medically unwell (for example, suffering from *unmada* of the Ayurvedic medical system), they would have been taken for medical treatment by their families; or if they were seen as 'possessed' or suffering from some supernatural affliction, they would have been helped by spiritual therapies.

Conclusions

It is noted in Chapter 2 that all cultural traditions include ideologies about 'madness' and about the 'mind', and that each cultural region developed somewhat different concepts around these matters. These differences (of tradition) set the stage for marked cultural diversity in how problems in the realm of the 'mind' are handled, and how concepts concerned with mental health and mental illness are conceptualized across the world. Although noting the dangers of generalizing when cultures are subject to change anyway, it is concluded in Chapter 2 that the western cultural tradition is characterized by a secular (non-spiritual) approach to mental health and illness while other, non-western, traditions either blend spiritual and bodily understandings or take a holistic approach to matters around mental health and illness. Also, it is noted there that not only the concepts of illness but also the ways in which illnesses are perceived (the explanatory models for illness)are different across cultural traditions (Kleinman, 1980); and boundaries between health and disease, and between mind and body, are drawn in different ways in different cultures. Clearly, these traditional differences would have resulted in very different arrangements developing in different settings for identifying and providing help for problems of living, whether identified as illness or not. In other words, societies that would be considered equally 'developed' may well have had (and still do have) very different systems for dealing with the needs of their people vis-à-vis (what we call today) mental health and mental illness.

Prior to the era of colonization, people in Asia would have had access to a variety of medical agencies, mainly based on Ayurveda, Chinese traditional medicine or the unani-Arabic system. All these recognized some aspects of 'madness' as illness and others as spiritual or existential issues. Similar but different systems were operating in most of Africa and probably in pre-Columbian America. Hence, if problems were perceived as medical, it is likely that some form of indigenous medical help would have been sought and very likely obtained. But the likelihood is that remedies for most mental problems (in psychiatric terms) would have been sought in religious practices and/or healing systems accepted in the cultural tradition concerned and believed in (and probably effective) because of this.

5
Colonial Psychiatry

Imperialism is about power and authority while colonialism is about people acquiring territories belonging to others and then exploiting people living there, but not necessarily settling there in large numbers (see definitions in *Oxford English Reference Dictionary* by Pearsall and Trumble, 1995). Empire-building need not be a part of imperialism. In her classic book *Imperial Leather*, Ann McClintock (1995) points out: 'Since the 1940s the U.S. imperialism-without-colonies has taken a number of distinct forms (military, political, economic and cultural), some concealed, some half-concealed. The power of U.S. financial capital and huge multinational corporations to command the flows of capital, research, consumer goods and media information around the world can exert a coercive power as great as any colonial gunboat' (p. 13).

The first period of modern imperialism for empire-building and colonization took place after the voyages of Columbus across the Atlantic in 1492. Land-grabbing, sometimes with genocide, and massive settlement led to the formation of a largely English-speaking Euro-American bloc in North America. Transatlantic plunder and the slave trade gave British imperialism and, to a lesser extent, that of other European countries, the wherewithal to embark on its second period of imperialism resulting in the subjugation of large parts of Asia and Africa. Between the late eighteenth and mid-twentieth centuries, European nations such as the Netherlands, Belgium, France and England, mainly the last two, established their Asian and African colonies. Some parts of Asia and Africa escaped a full boots-on-the ground occupation, but both continents, in effect, faced imperial domination; for example, China, although never completely colonized, was forced to accept domination through the opium wars (that forced China to accept opium imported by British traders), resulting in destruction and pillage and cultural intrusion. Porter (2012) describes the 'peculiar nature of early British imperialism': Initially driven by 'settlement and trade', British imperialism soon became a capitalist venture for 'material gain' with individuals and private companies seeking to enrich themselves; and then came 'cultural imperialism' (p. 7). Various social and political changes were imposed on its colonies by European imperial power; for example, class structures, languages, religious systems and political arrangements were imposed, destroying indigenous social organizations and so justifying (to their people at home) imperialism as a necessary part of fulfilling the 'white man's burden' (so-called after the title of a poem by Rudyard Kipling) to civilize and uplift allegedly primitive [sic] peoples.

Unlike the British approach, French imperialism was 'cultural' from the start although that did not prevent wealth extraction for the benefit of homeland France. France's overt purpose was to 'civilize' the natives by Europeanizing them culturally. Dispossession of native people and settlement of Europeans led to cultural and political extensions of Europe being established in far-away places such as Australia and New Zealand repeating the earlier imperialism of the seventeenth and eighteenth centuries in America. And with this colonialism came the age of economic underdevelopment of Asia and Africa wherever large European settlement was not established; and the suppression of indigenous cultures, including medical and other healing systems, literature, languages and the arts. It was mainly through cultural imperialism and its consequences on people's mindsets and expectations that Britain and France were able to police and govern large populations of Asian and African people for such a long time. It should be noted that the colonizers introduced services, such as transport systems, for example railways, which helped harness raw products in the colonies for export to Europe and set up European systems of education and healthcare available to natives as well as European expatriates. This is the background in which European colonizers, through its civil servants and, latterly, its western educated local elites, introduced *colonial psychiatry*.

A chapter on colonial psychiatry ideally should describe the problems of living encountered by ordinary people during colonial times and how, and to what extent, psychiatry affected them through the services it established. However, we do not have the sources for delving into all that, nor for examining conditions in many colonies, such as those held by the Portuguese and Spanish colonizers. In fact, I have selected for this chapter colonies where the sort of information I require was easily available in the literature, except that I left out colonies that were settled by significant numbers of Europeans, such as Australia and South Africa.

Hence, this chapter describes briefly the practice of psychiatry as introduced in some British and French colonies in Asia and Africa; and then, using this information, explores what the mental health scene might have been in those colonies for the native populations, and what deductions about the people there were drawn by colonialists who researched (in their own peculiar ways) the field of mental health as they saw it. I draw on studies of colonial psychiatry published in English, especially the books by Jock McCulloch (1995) on British colonies in Africa, Richard Keller (2007a) on French North Africa, and James Mills (2000) and Waltraud Ernst (2010) on British India, information being added to by bits and pieces from various other sources including my own observations in Sri Lanka in the dying days and immediate aftermath of colonialism.

My aim in this chapter is primarily to explore how people in the colonies, the natives, rather than expatriates, may have been affected by colonial psychiatry, especially in terms of how they used (if at all) the psychiatric services provided by colonizers, and what other ways they had at the time (of colonization) for supporting people with psychosocial problems and people seen as mad or insane. I try to avoid depicting the history of the colonized purely from the perspective of the West and I try to critique, rather than repeat, racist literature that colonial psychiatry produced in the shape of theories about the psychology of natives that some European professionals practising in the colonies produced. For example, the literature on psychiatry in East African British colonies are interspersed with opinions and 'research' carried out by Europeans such as H. L Gordon and J. C. Carothers, both superintendents of Mathari Mental Hospital in Nairobi (Kenya) (Mahone, 2007), describing what they called 'mental capacity' of Africans (Gordon, 1934) and the 'African Mind' (Carothers, 1953, 1972). Before some concluding remarks, there is a brief survey of how the writings and observations made in the colonies affected the construction of psychiatric and psychological knowledge *for the West* and how it may have contributed to the 'culture' of psychiatry itself and thence the experience of ethnic minorities in UK and France in the postcolonial era (Chapter 7).

Indian subcontinent

The countries that comprise modern India, Pakistan, Bangladesh, Myanmar (Burma) and Sri Lanka were all part of the British Empire. To cut a long story short, the British in effect took over much of what became British India (now India, Pakistan and Bangladesh) from the Mughals and added non-Mughal South India, Burma and Sri Lanka (calling it Ceylon) to its possessions. Then, populations in these areas had psychiatry introduced to them through the inauguration of asylums fashioned on British lines. The detaining of people in an institution because they were 'mad' was not consistent with the traditions and cultures of the area and certainly not the custom during Mughal rule in India. Although there were hospitals in Mughal India, there is no evidence that they catered for people considered 'mentally ill' or 'mad' as Islamic hospitals in the western part of the Islamic Empire undoubtedly did (Dols, 1992) (Chapter 2). In 1795, the British government in India established an institute for detaining 'mad' sepoys (Indian native soldiers employed by European agencies) in Bengal (Mills, 2000). Lunatic asylums were established in Bombay, Madras and Calcutta, the former two (unlike the one in Calcutta) admitting both Europeans and Eurasians (people of mixed European and native heritage). Also, 'native lunatic asylums' were established in various locations. According to Ernst (2010) all the asylums became overcrowded and priority for admission was '[perceived] danger to the community at large rather than their state of mind' especially in the case of native Indians (p. 37). But most Europeans deemed to be suffering from lunacy were repatriated to England as soon as possible—mainly to Pembroke House in Hackney (London).

In 1858, soon after direct rule from London replaced *ad hoc* rule by the East India Company with its own army of (mainly) sepoys, the British government in India drew up a legal framework for compulsorily detaining Indians deemed 'mad' by government agents (usually the police or army), and embarked on 'two decades of unprecedented activity in providing buildings to contain those the British encountered as "mad" in the Indian population' (Mills, 2000, p. 12). This was the nearest India, or indeed any part of Asia or Africa, got to Europe's large-scale confinement of lunatics—'the great confinement' (Foucault, 1967, p. 38)—noted in Chapters 2 and 3 as a highly significant event in European history that had a profound impact on how mental health and illness came to be seen in European culture. And, fortunately for India, the imposition of asylums more or less came to an end in 1880 at which time only about 2,750 patients were incarcerated in asylums in the whole of India and the numbers may well have fallen by 1990 (Mills, 2000). In contrast, in Germany, no less than one in every 500 of the population was confined in a lunatic asylum in 1911, and in England in 1909, asylum inmates were 3.7 per thousand population (Shorter, 1997).

The first asylum in Sri Lanka was not opened until 1847 and had just 47 patients (Uragoda, 1987). And in 1896, the only asylum in the country housed a mere 586 patients (Report of the Superintendent of Medical Services, 1896). But the asylum numbers probably went up in Sri Lanka during the first half of the twentieth century. There were 1,830 patients in the Angoda Asylum when it opened in 1926 (Uragoda, 1987) and when I worked there in the early 1960s (12 years after Ceylon became politically independent), there were over 4,000 in what was the only psychiatric facility in the country at the time, indicating that psychiatry was not playing much of a role in Sri Lankan society even then. The situation in Burma (which fell into British hands in 1885) was not dissimilar to that in British India. The British government established allopathic hospitals but indigenous doctors called *se-seyas* provided most of the general health care right through the British occupation (Htwe, 2001). According to Khin-Maung-Zaw (1997) a psychiatric facility called 'prison for the insane' was set up close to the City Prison in Rangoon merely for housing people considered a 'public nuisance' and an asylum was opened in 1926 in a village called Tadagalay with 250 residents, although the numbers there soon rose to 1,000 (1997, p. 506). Neither attempted to provide any treatment; they were both for containment only. It was not until after independence in 1948 that a psychiatric hospital was established.

Impact on local people

Clearly, the people incarcerated in asylums of British colonies in Asia were a highly selected population, mainly people who came to the attention of police or other government authorities because their behaviour was reckoned to be instigated by 'madness' rather than criminality. According to Mills (2000), many of the inmates were found to smoke cannabis and so it was assumed that cannabis caused madness, the British being unaware that cannabis usage was as common in the general population as it was among people they considered to be 'mad'. Labels were given for different types of behaviour and it was these labels that were recorded, not the stories behind them. Asylum inmates were of course given diagnoses in line with practices in England—diagnoses such as amentia, dementia, acute and chronic mania and moral insanity—but significantly the uncertainty of diagnosis was often commented upon by some medical officers. Study of case notes of the time led Mills to conclude: 'The discourses [in the case notes] . . . all linked to power relations in the period, to the fantasies and projects of European bourgeois masculinity, to the colonial order, to the rise of the medical profession and so on' (p. 41).

Mills (2000) contrasts the style of buildings and general approach in (indigenous) Indian healing centres (of which there were many) with that of European asylums that the British introduced: 'The lunatic asylum sought to impose a *moral* system on the patient through isolation and inducing guilt within the individual. The Indian approaches [to problems seen as "mental" or "madness"] emphasized the need to reintegrate the individual and advocated group involvement in treatment' (p. 131). Consequently when Indians used the asylum for their relatives—although they rejected their use at first, later some did use the asylums for short periods of time—it was used for punishment, often of 'junior members of the family being committed by senior ones' (p. 138). But some asylums in the subcontinent may have served a different purpose for the local people: When I worked as a junior doctor in Sri Lanka in the 1960s, I observed that some people incarcerated in the asylum near Colombo during the latter years of British rule, and still there in the 1960s, had been brought there by relatives after attempts had been made unsuccessfully to help them in the community; although most had been brought there by the police and apparently been abandoned or rejected by their relatives.

It seems that asylums in the colonized Indian subcontinent were not seen as places for treatment, merely for permanent incarceration. Mills (2000) noted that, in contrast to what happened in ordinary hospitals and other medical establishments, 'subordinate staff [of Indian asylums] had considerable power in day-to-day routine of asylum administration' (p. 150). This tallies with my observations in Sri Lanka in the 1960s where unqualified workers (called 'attendants') wielded immense power over patients and indirectly over nursing staff at Angoda Mental Hospital, the only asylum in the whole country at the time. The few nurses and doctors who were officially in charge of Angoda were powerless to prevent the harsh treatment and exploitation of patients that was then rampant and had been for many years going back into the colonial period. In the 1960s, I noted that few people were brought to the mental hospital at Angoda (unless forcibly admitted by the police) or to the (few) psychiatric outpatient clinics that had cropped up by then. This reflected the fact that local people in Sri Lanka did not see psychiatric treatment as very helpful. The extent to which indigenous therapies and healing practices were being used in the case of people who would otherwise have been brought for psychiatric treatment was unclear (to me) but the impression was that most people who needed help for (what I had learned in UK to recognize as) depression and psychoses were able to live in the community without causing undue concern mostly because they had some sort of help, be it religious healing or support of religious leaders, indigenous medical therapy or support of family and friends. It was possible, indeed likely, that people who were behaviourally uncontrollable (and these days liable to be diagnosed as suffering from acute psychosis or mania) were forcibly restrained in their homes but this was a very rare occurrence in Ceylon (as Sri Lanka was known at the time). So (in the early 1960s), either 'psychosis' (as an illness) was rare; people who may be diagnosed as 'psychotic' were accessing services that dealt positively with their problems; or such people were considered somewhat 'difficult', at worst a variant of normal human beings who did not require any special attention.

The Indian subcontinent (which formed the bulk of the British Empire) has always had a large number of healing centres connected with religious bodies. I was aware in the 1960s that many people in Sri Lanka, preferred to access healing therapies that were offered at Buddhist temples for problems identified as 'madness'. Also, some people who could afford it would seek the help of people called *aduras* (see Perera and Hettiarachchi, 2011), inaccurately described by westerners as 'exorcists' (Kapferer, 1991, p. 370), to arrange indigenous healing processes; or visit one of the many places where healing took place. But since the 1970s, psychiatric services have been developed gradually across the country and the custom now (1980s onwards), when someone is seen as possibly needing psychological-type medical help, is for the person concerned, with his/her relatives, to seek a plurality of services with a range of different approaches (see Chapter 4).

French North Africa

North Africa had been a part of a thriving Islamic Empire between the tenth to the thirteenth centuries. It was there that the foundations were laid for modern science (Masood, 2009) and where hospitals for people diagnosed with 'mental illness' (mainly melancholia) were first established (Chapters 2 and 3). Once the Empire, ruled by Caliphs in Bagdad and Cordoba, began to disintegrate and go downhill socially and economically, local rulers emerged, then the (Muslim) Ottomans and Mughals, and finally most of the region was occupied and exploited by European powers, Britain dominating the eastern regions (Egypt, Palestine, Iraq), and the French grabbing the western parts together with what remained of the Empire of Mali and neighbouring regions. The area colonized by the French was known as the Maghreb, comprising modern-day Algeria, Morocco and Tunisia. Colonization started with occupation of Algeria in the 1830s, leading on to the take-over of Tunisia (as a 'protectorate', but a colony in all but name) in 1881 and Morocco soon after that. Officially, the French incorporated the colonized regions as 'Departments' (provinces) of France itself but in effect—for the natives of the area, though perhaps not the French settlers—they were *de facto* colonies akin to British colonies in Asia and Africa.

Keller (2007a) describes how the French rulers of the Maghreb found that the *māristāns* (Islamic mental hospitals dating from the tenth century—see Chapter 2), had by the late nineteenth century fallen into 'a state of decadence' being no more than mere warehouses where people were kept in wretched misery (p. 34) in conditions which were even worse than those in the asylums of Europe. In Algeria, the French proceeded to suppress the *māristāns* and arranged for transport of people deemed insane to metropolitan asylums in France, and established dispensaries (outpatient clinics) and social service units. However, protests about public safety posed by un-hospitalized patients and the demands of European settler community for security led to institutions for 'the insane' being built in the Maghreb itself. From the 1930s, a series of institutions were opened that were planned from the outset as psychiatric hospitals rather than asylums (Keller, 2007b); moreover, dispensaries and social service units, not the hospital, formed the hub of a system to deliver psychiatric treatment, something far head of systems anywhere in the western world at the time. The first psychiatric hospital was established at Blida in 1938, later made famous by the fact that Frantz Fanon (see Macey, 2000) arrived there in 1947 and reformed its ways of working (McCulloch, 1983). Psychiatry in the Maghreb under the leadership of Professor Porot (see below) eagerly took up somatic 'treatments' considered experimental at best in France. In the 1940s ECT (electroconvulsive therapy or 'electroshock') became the 'bedrock of therapy in the Maghreb' and Professor Porot performed over 200 lobotomies between 1947 and 1954 (Keller, 2007b, pp. 29–30). By 1955, Blida, with its capacity of less than 1000 beds, held over 2000 patients (McCulloch, 1995). It is not clear how much of the psychiatric facilities were used voluntarily by native people of the Maghreb but clearly they had alternatives in their own indigenous systems to turn to (see below).

Impact on people of the Maghreb

During the height of the Islamic Empire (that lasted from the tenth to thirteenth centuries), a sophisticated health system was clearly in place in North Africa. People with problems identified as 'mental', mainly as melancholia, were taken care of by a medical system based on the *mārīstāns* that was partly derived from Greek medicine (see Chapter 2) almost certainly backed by systems of healing in the community—an arrangement described by Graham (1967) as a 'union of science and religion' (p. 47). Unlike the situation in the Indian subcontinent described earlier, the social and political structures including the hospital system had declined prior to French colonization of the Maghreb. It would seem that local people did not take to French asylum psychiatry however much it may have suited people of French origin, the settlers. In his book *Colonial Madness; Psychiatry in French North Africa*, Keller (2007a) writes:

Where French institutional psychiatry saw the asylum and its practices (including water treatments, work therapy, sedation, and confinement itself) as a panacea for a range of disorders, North African Muslims coped with mental illness in a number of ways. Many in the Maghreb recognized no distinction between illnesses of the mind and those of the body; the pluralism that obtained in much of North African medicine [and in Asia and Africa generally] therefore marked approaches to mental as well as physical disorder. Although the tradition of Avicennian [Greek] medicine based on theory of humours that had prevailed in the court culture of many medieval Islamic cities remained influential in those circles into the early modern period (and in some sectors to the present), by the late nineteenth and early twentieth centuries this tradition had largely given way to positivist medicine among the ruling elites of Morocco and Tunisia, as well as many Algerians. Among the urban poor in rural areas, however, the early modern period had witnessed the rise of the *marabouts*, or spiritual healers (from the Arabic *m'rabit*, or 'man connected to God') and cults of saints, which constitute a significant challenge to both humoral and positivist medical traditions [the positivist limits knowledge to what we can observe and measure], and which remain a primary source of healing for many contemporary North African Muslims. (pp. 25–26, italics in original)

The healers that most ordinary people in the Maghreb frequented practised exorcisms, spiritual healing of various sorts and other treatments delivered either in the community or the homes of the people deemed insane. But from Keller's account, it seems doubtful that this

healing catered adequately for people who were severely disturbed
behaviourally:

> For the chronically or violently ill and for those without the means
> to seek spiritual forms of healing, treatment was both more limited
> and more severe. Families often kept their insane relative locked in
> the home to protect them from themselves and others. For those
> who proved uncontrollable in the home, however, and those with-
> out family resources, the standard response was confinement in the
> *māristāns*. (p. 26, italics in original)

It seems that, although transfer to (European) asylums/mental hospitals
was theoretically available and there were European-style asylums in the
Maghreb itself, these facilities were mostly for the settlers.

Writing about the times towards the end of French colonialism
and the Algerian war of independence, Fanon (1965) commented:
'Western medical science, being part of the oppressive system, has
always provoked in the native an ambivalent attitude' (p. 121). Certainly overt racist thinking was common among French doctors in
charge of the institutions in the Maghreb; for example, Algerian psychiatrists (of French origin) made much of theories that connected
mental illness and criminality with 'both Islamic cultural traditions and
their suppositions about physical anomalies in North Africans' brains
structure', propositions that were 'the target of Frantz Fanon's outrage'
(Keller, 2007b, p. 25). From what Fanon wrote and the fact that he
resigned from his post as a psychiatrist to join the Algerian liberation
movement, it is likely that the French system of psychiatry was not
favourably received by people of the Maghreb and probably rarely used
voluntarily.

British Africa

Systematic exploration of Africa by Europeans and penetration by
Christian missionaries took place all through the nineteenth century,
accompanied by European countries taking charge of vast tracts of land
and the people living there. And then in 1884–1885, the Berlin conference of colonial powers agreed the borders of territories in Africa
that were shared out among them, legitimizing in European minds the
right for white nations to govern black Africans (and take their land).
'If the years 1880–1900 were broadly those of conquest.... the decades
1900–1920 may reasonably defined as the "period of pacification"

during which installation of colonial rule [cutting across tribal and cultural loyalties] was made complete' (Davidson, 1984, pp. 273–4). The British colonial Empire in Africa lasted until the 1960s when a wave of nationalist movements led to a series of independent African nations emerging, beginning with Ghana in 1957. The largest and most rewarding (to Britain) of its African colonies was Nigeria; the others included Uganda, Kenya, Gold Coast (later Ghana) and Rhodesia (later Zimbabwe), Malawi, Tanzania and Zambia. I can merely give a brief overview of psychiatry in some of these colonies in order to derive an impression of what local people may have thought of the system introduced by colonialists and what sort of help they may have accessed during colonial times for problems which today we call mental illness.

The first asylum in the British West Africa was established in Sierra Leone in 1844, followed by Accra Lunatic Asylum in Gold Coast 1888 and Yaba Asylum in Nigeria in 1906 (Patterson, 1981). Later, Mathari Hospital near Nairobi (Kenya) was established as the main asylum in East Africa. According to Law (2011) the lunatic asylum was 'the defining facility of colonial psychiatry [in Africa]' (p. 34); but there is a lack of information on the experiences of people who were incarcerated in asylums. According to McCulloch (1995) an official review of services in Nigeria in 1955 carried out by J. C. Carothers, a British psychiatrist stationed in Nairobi (Kenya), found that only the 'vagabond mad' (p. 32) came to the attentions of colonial authorities. For such people, there were small units administered by local authorities: In the south, they were 'prison lunatic asylums' attached to prisons; and in the north, they were asylums consisting of mud or clay cells where at best a doctor visited the inmates weekly (p. 32).

Interestingly, the report by Carothers (quoted by McCulloch, 1995) described two types of indigenous hospitals available to natives in Nigeria: The ones in townships consisted of huts which were 'stuffy and dark' and had doctors who were 'self-taught' and charged fees for treatment (with chants and prayers). However, African hospitals of the 'developed type' in rural areas were very different. In these, the doctor in charge was invariably an old man who had studied general medicine for five years, usually under his father, and had then spent a further three years specializing in 'psychiatry'. Such hospitals resembled traditional villages with a large number of individual huts in which the better-behaved stayed, sometimes with relatives who acted as guardians. There was a refractory ward for the acute cases, and people so designated were chained to logs or pinioned by their ankles. Treatment consisted of herbal remedies and the performance of rituals. When they had recovered sufficiently, the inmates were set to work producing food or tending animals, such labour being performed in the place of a fee. According to McCulloch (1995) 'Carothers found that relations between doctors and their patients [in rural hospitals] were excellent and concluded that the work of such physicians was necessary, humane and intelligent' (pp. 31–2).

Treatment available in European-style asylums was sparse: 'Before 1938, there was virtually no treatment provided' in any colonial (Sub-Saharan) asylum; and 'when treatment began it was in the form of convulsive therapy' (McCulloch, 1995, p. 43). Clearly ECT (electroplexy) was extensively used in African asylums and for all one knows, the situation may not have changed that much. A commission to inquire into conditions at Ingutsheni, an asylum near Bulawayo (Rhodesia), heard in 1942 that the death rate among African inmates was five to six per month mainly due to indiscriminate use of ECT and that practically 'all African inmates were given ECT, regardless of their physical or mental condition' (p. 38).

Clearly indigenous treatment (for what we call 'mental illness') was widely available during colonial times in Nigeria and other African colonies and accessed by local people. In the Gold Coast (now Ghana), Field (1960) described Ashanti shrines where people with 'fear and guilt frenzies' and people who were (as she put it) 'indistinguishable from classical schizophrenics' benefitted from attending (p. 1045); and another shrine where most of the devotees attending it could be diagnosed as suffering psychotic depression (Field, 1958). Even today, indigenous therapies are still much more popular in Ghana than are allopathic therapies (Ae-Ngibise *et al.*, 2010; Read, 2012) and probably more effective—or at least there is no evidence that they are not. Among the Yoruba (of Western Nigeria) concepts of health and medicine 'intertwined culturally with religion' and the people who provided individualized mental health care were predominantly indigenous healers. These healers used herbs and incantations (chants with ritualistic traditions) to perform cures (Law, 2011, p. 5). Indigenous healers passed on their knowledge verbally to their apprentices and, since what they pass on is based not just on what they had learned but what they found to be effective, the indigenous system was constantly being updated through experience.

Margaret Field (1960), a doctor and anthropologist working for the British colonial office in the Gold Coast in the 1950s, clearly did not think much of the one asylum available in the Gold Coast at the time.

[The] majority of chronic schizophrenics in rural districts are treated with such patience and sustained kindness by their relatives and tolerance by their neighbours that a prognosis for their recovery is probably better than it would be were they herded with other patients in under-staffed mental hospitals. If they have phases of destructive violence or of wandering off into the bush they are usually locked up or fettered to a log during these phases but released at the earliest possible moment. (pp. 453–4)

Impact on Africans

What is clear from the information available of colonial psychiatry in British colonies in Africa is that, overall, the numbers of people held in European-style asylums were very small compared to numbers in Europe. According to McCulloch (1995) they amounted to no more than 1,171 persons in 1960. Clearly, as in India, there had been no 'great confinement' (see earlier this chapter) in sub-Saharan Africa in spite of colonization and attempts at imposition of psychiatry. Nor, it would seem, did the native people accept the asylums as places for treatment of illness or 'madness'. It is very likely that asylum-psychiatry introduced in sub-Saharan Africa by British colonizers was peripheral to the mental health needs of people in the area. The asylums may well have served a social control function allied to colonial subjugation but certainly not a therapeutic one. Most Africans in British colonies who required help for (what we call) mental health problems would have accessed, if they accessed any agencies outside the family and community, religious healing and indigenous medicine. And it seems highly likely that these were available widely and used fairly extensively.

Contributions to psychiatric knowledge

Colonial psychiatry in India did not impact very much on the diverse cultural roots of that region and clearly had little effect on medical or non-medical healing practices in the subcontinent during colonial times. And, very little in the way of observations and hypotheses about native people made by British psychiatrists working in British India have come through as 'knowledge' incorporated into psychiatry. It should be noted that Carl Jung hypothesized about the Indian mind, having visited India during colonial times and drawn on Indian philosophy for some of his theories of psychological functioning. Jung (1939) observed a 'very characteristic defect in the Indian character... [namely]... deception' (p. 524). This was mildly racist but it was his theories about Africans that have attracted much attention for their overt racist connotations. On his return from the USA in the 1930s, Jung proposed his theory of 'racial infection'—'a very serious mental and moral problem wherever a primitive race outnumbers the white man':

> Now what is more contagious than to live side by side with a rather primitive people? Go to Africa and see what happens. When the effect is so very obvious that you stumble over it, then you call it 'going black'... The inferior man exercises a tremendous pull upon civilized beings who are forced to live with him, because he fascinates the inferior layers of our psyche, which has lived through untold ages of similar conditions.
>
> (Jung, 1930, p. 196)

It is outside the scope of this book to discuss this and other racist ideas that Jung proposed—well covered elsewhere (Dalal, 1988; Fernando, 2003).

Two British figures stand out in the colonial project to impose psychiatry in East Africa (Mahone, 2007): H. L. Gordon and J. C. Carothers. The former, a medical doctor who was posted to Mathari (Mental) Hospital in Nairobi postulated 'some remarkable facts [*sic*] concerning the brains of East African natives'... [namely]... low degree of mentality... constituting.... social danger' (Sequeira, 1932, p. 581). He was followed at Mathari Hospital by J. C. Carothers who produced a large body of psychiatric-psychological publications on Africans. These two doctors, who essentially proposed that African brains were underdeveloped with malfunctioning of the frontal lobes, have in post-colonial times been dubbed the 'leaders of scientific racism in the African colonies' (Mahone, 2007, p. 45). Carothers (1951) echoed Gordon's view that Africans were deficient in frontal lobe function and proposed a 'resemblance between the African and the leucotomised European' (p. 12). (Leucotomy was another name for lobotomy when parts of the brain were surgically destroyed—referred to in Chapter 3.) Carothers was widely recognized as a leading theoretician on the psychology of Africans. When commissioned by the World Health Organization (WHO) to write a report on Africans he produced *The African Mind in Health and Disease* (Carothers, 1953). Here, Carothers wrote about the lack of depression among Africans because (he claimed) they lacked 'a sense of responsibility'; described their madness as a form of 'primitive psychosis'; and claimed that 'the resemblance of the leuco-tomised European patient to the primitive African is, in many cases, complete' (p. 157).

Like their British counterparts in sub-Saharan Africa, French psychia-trists came up with similar observations about the psychology of North African people. The Algiers school of French psychiatry was founded by Professor Antoine Porot who achieved fame for 'research' in 'ethno-psychiatry'. According to Keller (2007b), in 1918 Porot 'framed the "North African" as inherently puerile and incapable of coping with the realities of modern civilization' (p. 25); and then in 1925 produced spurious data showing the African mind as being 'primitive, crimi-nally impulsive, and intellectually feeble' (p. 18). Fanon (1967) quotes Porot to have stated in 1935 at the Congress of Mental Specialists and Neurologists that 'the native of North Africa, whose superior and corti-cal activities are only slightly developed, is a primitive creature whose life, essentially vegetative and instinctive, is above all regulated by his diencephalon [developmentally primitive part of the brain]' (p. 243). Porot's work, together with 'observations' [*sic*] by other French psychi-atrists working in North Africa on 'primitive mentalities' and 'criminal impulsiveness' of North Africans, became incorporated into the 'disci-pline of ethno-psychiatry [that] informed education and professional discrimination against Muslims, shaped discourse about immigration into France, and provided the essential background for the French army's psychological warfare programs during the Algerian struggle for independence' (Keller, 2007a, p. 7). It is likely that ideas in French 'ethno-psychiatry' may influence psychiatric practice in France today vis-à-vis French citizens of North African origin living in France. How-ever, this is not a topic that has been researched or discussed at all in contemporary literature, unlike the case of UK where the discourse on racism in British psychiatric practice is well established (Bhui, 2002; Fernando, 2003, 2010; and Chapter 7).

Conclusions

The colonial era of exploitation of people and resources of Asia and Africa that set western nations up as the rich part of the world was a time when European powers imposed their own cultural forms and institu-tions on the people of the regions they dominated. One such institution was European asylum psychiatry.

Earlier chapters (especially Chapters 2 and 4) indicate that what is called 'mental health' in the West is generally seen in non-western cultures in terms of balance of body-mind-spirit. Also, compared to what happened in the West (Chapter 3), there was little in the way of medicalization of social, spiritual and emotional problems in the non-western world. For these reasons, and also because colonial systems were often permeated by racism, the impact of colonial psychiatry is likely to have been minimal in terms of providing services for help and support of people who (in psychiatric terms) suffered from mental health problems. Most native people in the European colonies continued to look to indigenous and traditional systems for help for problems of madness and the sort of problems (social, behavioural and emotional) that may be interpreted in psychiatric terms as 'mental illness'. The impact of colonial psychiatry is summarized in Table 5.1. On the whole, people of the (British) Indian subcontinent, the (French) Maghreb and (British) sub-Saharan Africa did not take up the system of psychiatric treatment that the colonial powers introduced. Native people of the colonies continued to look to indigenous systems of help and support for (what could be termed mental health problems) although colonial powers underdeveloped these and sometimes actively suppressed them. Significantly, there was no 'great confinement' (massive institutionalisation) of people designated as 'mentally ill' as there was in Europe. The contribution to psychiatric knowledge [*sic*] from colonial psychiatry is significant for multicultural western societies in the twenty-first century because, together with other racist psychiatric literature from the times of slavery (see Chapter 3), so-called 'observations' on Asians and Africans made by colonial psychiatrists have fed into stereotypes and myths about people who are seen as non-white, especially black people, and these contribute to institutional racism in psychiatric practice in modern times—a matter that is referred to in Chapters 6 and 7.

Colonialism left developing countries an unenviable legacy in the field of mental health. Indigenous systems for mental health were left underdeveloped or actively suppressed and ex-colonial countries were left with underfunded and oppressive asylums in the European style. Yet the greatest problem for mental health development may well be a

Table 5.1 Impact of colonial psychiatry

Underdevelopment of indigenous systems
European-style asylums with little 'treatment'
No 'great confinement' (as in Europe)
Asylums used for incarceration rather than treatment
Contributions to psychiatric knowledge

---

more subtle psychological legacy. Imperialism and colonization meant much more than European physical presence and the exploitation of their natural resources and indigenous labour; it entailed the permeation of a particular mindset of patronising arrogance in the European consciousness towards 'the natives' and their cultures and the instillation of what Homi Bhabha (1994), drawing on the work of Frantz Fanon (1952, 1959, 1961), calls 'the colonial condition' in (colonized) Asians and Africans:

> If the order of Western historicism is disturbed in the colonial state of emergency, even more deeply disturbed is the social and psychic representation of the human subject. For the very nature of humanity becomes estranged in the colonial condition and from that 'naked declivity' it emerges, not as an assertion of will nor as an evocation of freedom, but as an enigmatic questioning.
>
> (Bhabha, 1994, pp. 41–2)

The patronising arrogance of the West, the 'we know best' approach, still appears in dealings between nations divided by geo-political power structures of the world; and, as Homi Bhabha (1994) puts it, 'a range of culturally and racially marginalized groups... [struggle today with]... the crucial engagement between mask and identity, image and identification... [with the vital question for today's world]... How can the human world live its difference? How can a human being live Other-wise?' (pp. 63–4).

What actually happened in the post-colonial era will be considered in the next part of the book (Chapters 6, 7 and 8); and possible ways forward in mental health development in LMICs in the Chapter 10.

Part III

Psychiatry and Mental Health after the Second World War: Exporting Psychiatry to the Global South

There were many cultural and social changes both in the Global North and the Global South following the fall of the European empires soon after the end of the Second World War. The three chapters of this part of the book describe the serious problems in the Euro-American system of psychiatry and look closely at the sociopolitical context of neo-liberalism and the power of multinational corporations in which bio-medical psychiatry is marketed across the world.

6
Medication Revolution and Emerging Discontents

The centres of research and progress in psychiatric theory and practice from the 1950s onwards were in the US–UK axis, particularly the USA. As the asylums were phased out, the great medication revolution—no less significant than the 'great confinement [of lunatics in asylums]' (Foucault, 1967, p. 38) described in Chapter 3—gradually took hold. The end result was that standard psychiatric practice became basically a matter of matching therapy, usually medication, to diagnoses based on nosology agreed in Europe and the USA after the end of the Second World War (WWII)—*ICD-6 Classification of Mental and Behavioural Disorders* (ICD-6) (WHO, 1948) or *Mental Disorders: Diagnostic and Statistical Manual* (DSM-I) (APA, 1952). As a psychiatrist in the British National Health Service (NHS) from the early 1960s onwards, I was part of a changing system, working, at first, in asylums, then at a teaching hospital in central London and then in a psychiatric unit in a general hospital and in the adjoining community.

This chapter starts by discussing the changes in psychiatric practice during the 1960s to the 1990s and what they felt like at the level of clinical practice; and how the changes led to the current system of psychiatric practice. From being, during asylum times, a rather muddled amalgamation of social care and control with minimal focus on treatment of illness, psychiatry developed into a medical discipline confident that it was providing remedies for mental illness and emotional disturbances, whatever the cause; and for good measure throwing in so-called 'disorders' of personality. The social and cultural elements of mental illness got pushed to the sidelines; the ability to make specific diagnoses became the standard by which the expertise of psychiatrists was judged by their peers and later by the general public. The psychiatric profession as a body (though not all psychiatrists) sold psychiatry, and the general public in the UK largely bought it, as a scientific medical discipline with a view on any personal problem traceable theoretically to individual human behaviour and/or distress or suffering that did not have an easily discernible explanation in bodily (somatic) terms. In much of this chapter, I refer to users of services as 'patients' as was the habit until the mid or late 1990s when the rising service user movements in UK and North America brought about a change.

The 1960s and 1970s in England was a time of immigration from Asia, Africa and the Caribbean. The melting pot of USA society was shown up as the charade that it always was and, in UK, issues of race and culture began to surface, not just in society at large but in the field of mental health service delivery and psychiatric practice. The USA saw the civil rights movement of the 1960s, and racial tensions in England in the 1970s led to 'race riots' in several British cities in the early 1980s. This chapter refers to the problems that surfaced in UK as 'ethnic issues' arising at the interface between mental health service provision and the cultural and racial diversity in British society. It outlines the serious questions that started to be asked in the late 1980s and 1990s, about the practice of psychiatry itself; not just by people from non-western backgrounds concerned at its Eurocentric and possibly racist nature but by society in general and, later, even by many practitioners within the discipline itself. In addition, movements within psychiatry itself, such as the so-called 'anti-psychiatry movement' (Laing, 1967; Laing and Esterson, 1964) and British transcultural psychiatry (represented for example in books by Fernando, 1988; Littlewood and Lipsedge, 1982; and Rack, 1982) challenged traditional (western) views of mental illness and its treatment; and movements among ex-patients (for example in the USA by Chamberlin, 1978) who defined themselves as survivors of the psychiatric system became increasingly influential. All this was the precursor to the questioning of psychiatric practice today (2013) on both sides of the Atlantic, not least by many professionals working in mental health services (see below). Finally, the chapter concludes by summarizing the current state of psychiatric practice and mental health service provision as full of discontents and anomalies, so much so that one could say that both psychiatry itself and mental health service provision are both in a state of crisis.

Changes from the 1960s onwards

As the enormity of the Nazi racist crimes of the 1940s became known, there was a revulsion against locking people up for being 'different' and a feeling for individual human rights in Europe and North America. Also, interest grew post-war in both UK and USA in the impact of social environment on mental health and illness (Faris, 1967; Faris and Dunham, 1939; Felix and Bowers, 1948; Hollingshead and Redlich, 1958) and, in some limited settings often promoted by charismatic and dedicated individuals, social and community psychiatry seemed to offer a new way for organizing services. Experimental systems such as the 'colony for the insane' at Gheel in Belgium, Scottish hospitals offering 'family care', and in the 1950s, social rehabilitation units and therapeutic communities in mental hospitals, came on the scene (Shorter, 1997, pp. 229–34). I had the privilege of working at Claybury Hospital in north-east London where the 'therapeutic community approach' for the general run of psychiatric patients admitted to hospital was pioneered (Shoenberg, 1972). And about the same time, 'crisis intervention' was pioneered as an alternative to hospital admission at Napsbury Hospital at St Albans (UK) (Scott, 1960).

In the late 1950s, a neuroleptic drug (neuroleptics act on the nervous system and include 'psychotropics' which affect the 'mind' by altering brain function), chlorpromazine, was tried out as a hypnotic but soon became something that seemed to subdue symptoms of mental illness (Delay *et al.*, 1952); and by 1954 it was being used clinically for mental illness (Healy, 1990). It is now clear that chlorpromazine was no more than a powerful tranquilizer that made people feel calm if they were highly aroused emotionally, but at the time it became popular (in the 1960s) this drug appeared to 'treat' mental illness, especially schizophrenia. Soon, this and other similar drugs were marketed as 'antipsychotics'; and drugs came on the scene marketed as 'anti-depressants', and later some as 'anxiolytics' (anti-anxiety drugs). In studying the effect of these medications on brain-chemistry, various theories were constructed about chemical causes of the illnesses that Kraepelin and others after him had constructed. Although no specific abnormalities of brain chemistry were found to be associated with any of these illnesses, the story took hold that mental illness was caused by 'chemical imbalance' in the brain. And these new types of drugs achieved the reputation of curing mental illness. Many psychiatrists went along with this, some believing in it; moreover, it suited the profession in selling their trade, suited the pharmaceutical industry in making profits, and assured many people that psychiatry had specific medical treatments for mental illness.

The emptying of mental hospitals, de-institutionalization (Scull, 1977), began in England in the mid-1970s and accelerated in the 1980s and 1990s when the so-called era of community care came into being, replacing asylums. It is now clear that drug therapy had little to do with de-institutionalization (Eisenberg, 2000; Scull, 1984), although it may have helped later on in persuading doctors and the general public that it was safe to allow mental patients to live in the community. 'Decarceration was driven far more by fiscal concerns—the massive costs of running and replacing the traditional mental hospitals' (Scull, 2011, pp. 116–17). But the knowledge constructed at the time of bio-medical enthusiasm meant that the notion that mental illness, including depression and anxiety states, was caused by neuro-chemical disturbances was taught as gospel. By the mid-1960s, there was an air of optimism in Euro-America that psychiatry was in the throes of a revolution in treating mental illness with physical (mainly drug) remedies, apparently justifying the traditional Kraepelian ideology of genetic-biological causes of mental illness. When I was looking for trainee positions as a 'junior doctor' in psychiatry in the UK, I heard of the keen competition for jobs at what was (in the 1960s) considered a centre of excellence in 'scientific' psychiatry, the Institute of Psychiatry (IOP) in London. I recall that in the 1960s and 1970s, many clever, scientifically-minded people went into psychiatry and allied disciplines in teaching hospitals imagining that they were at the frontiers of medical science; and in the mid-1970s, there was no problem in filling posts in psychiatric units in General Hospitals that were coming on stream in the UK since psychiatry was now seen as a truly medical discipline.

Drift into drug-based psychiatry

Neuroleptic drugs marketed as 'anti-psychotics' and 'anti-depressants' indeed changed psychiatric practice dramatically in the 1960s and 1970s. When I worked at Claybury Hospital in the late-1960s and 1970s (see earlier), I saw how the 'therapeutic community' approach was being undermined by newer psychiatrists coming in with 'modern' (drug-based) ways of treatment and a faith in ECT (electroconvulsive therapy), deriding the practice of older psychiatrists who continued to look to more psychological approaches in treatment.

When in 1976 I was consultant in charge of an admission ward at a psychiatric unit in a District General Hospital (one of the first such units in England at Chase Farm Hospital, Enfield, Middlesex, UK), I tried to pursue some of the therapeutic community approaches (such as large group meetings) I had tasted at Claybury. This meant essentially discussing problems and their possible resolutions in 'community meetings' and seeing patients individually and in private (rather than in the traditional medical 'round' attended by a team of professionals). I was under a lot or pressure from younger staff to pursue (by then) the standard approach of interviewing patients on a ward round and then discussing their treatment with the staff, who then implemented the decisions. Gradually the discourse shifted into 'packages of treatment' and later these were linked to defining objective outcomes in the language of symptoms and diagnoses. The bi-weekly community meetings (an essential part of a therapeutic community approach in ward management) lapsed through non-attendance of staff. I was considered old-fashioned to resist the developing technological approach. And then came pressure to measure individual outcomes in terms of symptom reduction.

In my training in the early 1960s, I had learned that diagnoses were not that important and (when I was undergoing training) trainees were tested on their ability to produce formulations describing the life situations and problems that patients faced. But as I heard in the late 1970s and 1980s how trainees were being tested during their examinations— mainly about effects of drugs and knowledge of symptoms—I had to shift partly into teaching them how to get through examinations. I tried to balance both approaches by suggesting to trainees that they should list symptoms and make diagnoses but then leave that information aside and get on with getting to know their patients.

In the late 1970s, the pressure to make diagnoses in line with definitions in international classifications drove organizational systems set up in hospitals for 'managing' patients; and the pharmaceutical industry gradually became major players in the field of treating mental illness. When I was working as a consultant psychiatrist at Chase Farm Hospital Mental Health Unit in the 1980s, several members of staff wanted a pharmacist to attend the ward round; and I saw later that it was considered officially (by the Department of Health) to be good practice for a pharmacist (who never talked to the patients but knew about the effects of various drugs on brain chemistry) to advice on matching drugs to symptoms. Much later (in the late 1980s) when I was a member of an inspectorate (called the Mental Health Act Commission) many of my colleagues who inspected hospitals to monitor patient-care thought it only right that pharmacists should be closely involved in decision-making on treatment of patients; and these colleagues were mainly non-medical people like social workers, psychologists and people from the (lay) voluntary sector.

It was not just the culture of psychiatry that changed from the1970s onwards, but society in general gradually adopted ways of thinking set up by psychiatry during the medication revolution: Symptom control was the be-all and end-all of treatment for mental health problems and good psychiatric practice meant the ability to make clear diagnoses and administer drug remedies. This change in ways of thinking is a form of 'looping effect' described by Hacking (1995, 1999) whereby psychological and psychiatric categories and constructs that circulate in the wider world get internalized by individuals and shape their experiences and observations. I realized that the drug-based approach to treatment meant that it was not the patient who was being treated—it was the symptom(s) and/or the diagnosed illness; and this was becoming the norm in the NHS.

The diagnostic approach to describing a range of problems became increasingly popular in the 1970s and in the 1980s; and randomized controlled trials (of drug therapy), often sponsored by pharmaceutical companies, became the gold standard for research into treatment of psychiatric illness (Kirmayer, 2012). With this came the drive in psychiatry to adopt 'evidence-based medicine' (EBM) as the measure of good practice. This approach demands that decision-making vis-à-vis psychiatric treatment is based on best 'evidence'—defined as *research evidence* (not, for example, the evidence of people who use psychiatric services) and 'research' usually means deductions from 'quantitative data drawn from experimental studies, preferably randomized controlled trials [RCTs] or meta-analyses of these trials' (Gupta, 2007, p. 105). As psychiatric services became more available, the consumption of medication by the general public increased and influence of the pharmaceutical industry widened. By the mid-1980s, the bio-medical approach, focusing on medication and other physical interventions (such as ECT) became standard practice, superseding talking therapies (psychotherapy) which could not be quantified for research purposes and hence considered unscientific. And the pharmaceutical companies produced greater and greater varieties of (what they marketed as) 'anti-psychotics' and 'anti-depressants'. Quick diagnosis and specific treatment directed at symptoms and illness (rather than the patient and the problems (s)he faced) became the model for training. By the 1990s, use of drugs as specific treatments for mental illnesses, often conceptualized as purely brain diseases although given psychiatric (mental), not neurological (medical), diagnoses, became standard practice. The so-called anti-depressants flourished and *pari passu* the diagnosis of depression soared in popularity. The World Health Organization (WHO, 2012) forecasts that 'by 2030 depression will be the leading cause of disease burden globally' (WHO, 2012, p. 1), and the World Federation for Mental Health (WFMH) (2012) claims that depression (as an illness) is now a global crisis (2012, title page)—and that in a document made possible by grants from Lundbeck and Lilly, two pharmaceutical companies that manufacture medication marketed as antidepressants.

Biological hypotheses for schizophrenia and depression, based on the modes of chemical action on the brain of so-called 'anti-psychotics' and 'anti-depressants', and *not* on observed variations in brain chemistry in people diagnosed with the illnesses concerned, appeared in the 1960s and 1970s. Like many drugs promoted by pharmaceutical companies as remedies for schizophrenia and depression, these hypotheses too have multiplied since then. Although unproven, these chemical hypotheses for the causation of mental illness remain very much in the forefront of thinking about any problem seen as 'mental' or 'psychological' in origin or manifestation, not just within psychiatric circles but within society at large. 'Chemical imbalance' in the brain is now promoted in the public domain as the cause of many so-called mental health problems. One reason for this may be that neuroleptics do seem to suppress feelings and emotional states that are considered 'symptoms' of illness; in other words they are effective tranquillizers. The problem is that feelings and emotional states have become medicalized (constructed as medical issues) by psychiatric conditioning of society (yet another form of 'looping'—see earlier this chapter). But David Healy (1990), psychopharmacologist and professor of psychiatry in Wales, draws attention to other sociopolitical factors too being important for the ascendancy of biological hypotheses by comparing the current situation to that in the early twentieth century:

> But other factors seem [to be] suggested by the example of the adoption of morbid heredity and degeneration in French psychiatry precisely 100 years earlier [see Chapter 2]. At this time French psychiatrists were beset by problems. The public held them in low repute. The magistracy derided their claims to legal expertise. The profession was sharply divided along theoretical lines. The situation faced by psychiatry... 100 years later.
>
> (Healy, 1990, p. 67)

Collusion between psychiatry and pharma

It was in the USA that drug-based psychiatry really took off in a context of market forces. From the late-1980s, Kraepelian or 'neo-Kraepelian' thinking has dominated psychiatric practice, supported by the pharmaceutical industry (Pharma) producing newer and newer neuroleptic drugs marketed as specific remedies for the vast number of mental illnesses listed in successive editions of the (American) Diagnostic Statistical Manual (DSM): 'As psychiatry became a drug-intensive speciality, the pharmaceutical industry was quick to see the advantages of forming an alliance with the psychiatric profession' (Angell, 2011b, p. 4). Today (2013) drugs that affect neurological and mental activity are marketed directly and openly as remedies for a variety of human problems presented as 'illnesses'; and it is considered normal, correct practice for psychiatrists to turn to one or other drug (or often several together) as the treatment for practically any 'condition' they diagnose or even when they feel unable to make a specific diagnosis.

Changes in the fashion or style of diagnosing over the years are reflected in changes in successive editions of DSM. Whitaker (2010) points out that, while the first two editions of DSM, published in 1952 and 1968, reflected the Freudian view of mental illness (still the illness model but with a wider interpretation of what is illness compared to the narrow bio-medical one of German-British psychiatry), DSM-III published in 1980 was something quite different. It contained 256 diagnoses (as opposed to 182 in the previous version), but even more importantly, each diagnosis was defined by a list of symptoms with numerical thresholds for making the diagnosis. Diagnoses under DSM-III became more reliable in that agreement between clinicians increased but with no change in their lack of validity as representing 'illness'. Also, DSM-III provided a system which can be used for a tickbox exercise in making diagnoses for whatever purpose. The number of DSM-recognized illnesses has multiplied over the years: DSM-IV-TR (revised version of DSM-IV) (APA, 2000) contains 365 diagnoses. DSM 5 (APA, 2013) released in May 2013 after much contentious debate and opposition from service users, psychologists and many psychiatrists, takes this even further. And American practice inevitably spreads to UK and then the rest of Europe, although the official categorization of illness in Europe is supposed to be in line with ICD-10 (WHO, 1992) rather than the American DSM. But, even more serious is the power that DSM exerts in developing countries (Chapters 8 and 10). Further comments on DSM 5 appear in Chapter 11.

Some psychiatrists (for example, Kendell and Jablensky, 2003) have argued that psychiatric diagnosis may not be scientifically valid categories for identifying illness since they were defined in terms of syndromes (collections of symptoms), but are useful for clinical purposes on the grounds of utility: 'Many, though not all, of the diagnostic concepts represented by the categories of disorder listed in contemporary nomenclatures such as DSM-IV and ICD-10 are extremely useful to practising clinicians, and most clinicians would be hard put to cope without them' (p. 9). And more recently, in a debate about the effects on service provision (for people with mental health problems), David and Sartorius (2013) argue that the diagnostic framework ensures that resources are allocated appropriately because 'diagnosis provides boundaries' (2013, p. 21). The lesson from these arguments supporting the continued use of psychiatric diagnoses is that their use at the very least requires careful control by society at large; that the relevance of the 'illness model' (that is its usefulness) for a particular situation should be assessed before any diagnosis is actually made. However, the warnings implicit in these arguments about validity and utility cut little ice in ordinary psychiatric practice or in psychiatric research. The bulk of practising psychiatrists and researchers reify diagnosis as a 'thing' that is separate from the person receiving the diagnosis; and they carry on as if the use of diagnosis-based illness categories is fully justified; in many ways so far the general public seem to go along with this—but I guess not for long.

Critiques of bio-medical (western) psychiatry

It should be noted that dissenting voices objecting to the diagnostic approach to mental health emerged in the 1960s (when incidentally there were anti-establishment groups in many other fields too). In USA, Thomas Szasz (1962) in the *Myth of Mental Illness* and sociologists such as Thomas Scheff (1966) challenged the traditional biological view of mental illness. In Britain, similar views developed into the so-called anti-psychiatry movement led by Laing and Esterson (Cooper, 1970) (Laing himself denied being 'anti-psychiatry'); although this movement did not deny the mental illness, particularly schizophrenia, as an individual reality, it was perceived as a way of coping within families; essentially 'illness' seen as being caused by problems within families, use being made of concepts such as the 'double-bind' where people were caught up in states of psychological conflict (Bateson *et al.*, 1956). This movement led to the setting up of a residential establishment, Kingsley Hall, in the East End of London in the late sixties, its work being described vividly in *Two Accounts of a Journey Through Madness* (Barnes and Berke, 1971). Inspired by the work at Kingsley Hall, Loren Mosher, an American psychiatrist, set up Soteria House in 1971 in California; here people diagnosed as suffering schizophrenia were treated without the use of neuroleptics (Thomas, 2013). But all this was peripheral to mainstream of Euro-American psychiatric practice.

Much of the dissent within psychiatry in the 1970s and 1980s was submerged by what appeared as progress in the shape of increasing reliability in classifying 'mental illnesses' and increasing number of remedies being marketed for mental health problems, nearly always for diagnosable illnesses. An article by George Engel (1977) highlighted the movement within psychiatry 'to emulate its sister medical disciplines by finally embracing once and for all the [narrow] medical model of disease' (p. 129) and suggested instead that western medicine as a whole, including psychiatry, should adopt a 'biopsychosocial' (BPS) model to replace the reductionist approach: 'The boundaries between health and disease, between well and sick, are far from clear, and never will be clear, for they are diffused by cultural, social and psychological considerations' (p. 132). Although the BPS model was indeed taken up to guide theoretical exploration it was not taken up in clinical practice to any extent in psychiatry.

Transcultural critiques

The psychiatric approach to problems of living and the way mental health services are structured in general have been severely criticized in the UK since the early 1980s by people from non-western backgrounds who had settled in many parts of the country since the 1960s. Much of the critique was voiced through, and by, the movement called 'transcultural psychiatry' centred in the 1980s and 1990s on the Transcultural Psychiatry Society (TCPS) (UK) (see Bains, 2005; Fernando, 1988, 2003; Vige, 2008). The transcultural critique in UK has been largely around the Eurocentric nature of the medical model being used in psychiatric practice and (western) psychological theories, institutional racism in mental health services, racism within psychiatry itself and the criminalization within psychiatry, especially in its forensic services, of black and Asian people in the UK who present with serious social and personal problems often inappropriately attributed to 'mental illness' (Bhui and Olajide, 1999; Fernando, 1988, 1991, 2003, 2010; Fernando *et al.*, 1998; Littlewood and Lipsedge,1982, 1997; Rack, 1982).

The critiques from the transcultural psychiatry movement of the 1980s and 1990s fed into a movement that emerged within the psychiatric profession in the late 1990s, forming the 'Critical Psychiatry Network' (CPN) (http://www.criticalpsychiatry.co.uk/). The main thrust of CPN allied with a critical movement within clinical psychology is that psychiatric nosology is unscientific (Bentall, 2010; Boyle, 2002; Johnstone, 2000; Thomas, 1997) and that remedies that psychiatry puts up for these so-called illnesses do not work—that the 'chemical cure' is a 'myth' (Moncrieff, 2009, title page).

Bio-medical psychiatry depends on diagnosis based on a medical model of illness and hypotheses about the mind that developed in Europe over the past 300 years (Chapter 2). The so-called mental phenomena that psychiatry deals with look very much like the sort of things that societies regulate—or try to (Ingleby, 1982). The social construction of mental illness was shown up dramatically in the political abuses of psychiatry in the Soviet Union (Bloch and Reddaway, 1984) and the decision of the American Psychiatric Association in 1973 that homosexuality should cease to be an 'illness' (Bayer, 1981). In both instances, political forces coupled with discriminatory attitudes were shown to have determined the nature of what constituted illness. Similarly, racist considerations were clearly evident in the construction of two diagnostic categories reported in the United States at the time of slavery and described by Cartwright (1851) as peculiar to black people, namely the disease causing black slaves to run abscond from plantations and the disease that caused others to rebel (Chapter 3). The transcultural critiques of diagnosis and western models of mental illness and research (largely voiced in UK) are discussed in Chapter 7 and the racist tradition in psychiatry is discussed in Chapter 3.

Arguments challenging the relevance of EBM in psychiatric practice has emerged on both sides of the Atlantic. These concern the mismatch between clinical trials and realities of patient experience which is not captured by diagnoses (Faulkner and Thomas, 2002; Gupta, 2007; Healy, 2001; Thomas *et al.*, 2012). Kirmayer (2012) summarizes the objections to EBM from a transcultural viewpoint:

> (1) The diagnostic and conceptual frameworks used to pose questions, devise interventions, and determine outcomes in EBP [evidence-based practice] are themselves culturally determined and therefore potentially biased or inappropriate; and (2) Cultural communities may have 'ways of knowing' that do not rely on the kinds of observational and experimental measures and methods that characterize EBP. (p. 249)

Recent critiques in the USA

There has been considerable criticism in the USA during the early part of the twenty-first century, both about the use of medications and about the model of mental illness generally referred to as 'Kraepelian' or 'neo-Krapelian' (Donald, 2001). Reviewing three important books for the prestigious *New York Review of Books*, Marcia Angell (2011a), former editor of the prestigious *New England Journal of Medicine*, came to two significant conclusions. The books she reviewed were by Irving Kirsch (2009), a professor of psychology at the University of Hull; Robert Whitaker (2010), an investigative journalist; and Daniel Carlat (2010), a psychiatrist who practises in a Boston suburb. Angell's conclusions were that (a) Pharmaceutical companies 'that sell psychoactive drugs through various forms of marketing, both legal and illegal, have come to determine what constitutes a mental illness and how these disorders should be diagnosed and treated' (Angell, 2011a, p. 3); (b) it is now highly doubtful that 'mental illness is caused by a chemical imbalance in the brain' (2011a, p. 3); and (c) there is now convincing evidence that psychoactive drugs are not just useless but may actually cause harm. In a second article, discussing the DSM and the book by Carlat (2010), Angell (2011b) criticized damningly the collusion between the American Psychiatric Association and the pharmaceutical industry in spreading the use of psychoactive drugs in the American population, condemning 'the "frenzy" of diagnosis, the overuse of drugs with sometimes devastating side effects, and the widespread conflict of interests [of people involved in the trade of making diagnoses and providing drugs]' (2011b, p. 7).

In addition to the evidence produced in the books referred to, there has been a spate of other books and papers published in the 2000s, rejecting the concept of mental illness as a predominantly biological issue (for example, Bentall, 2010); critical of the activities of the pharmaceutical industry (for example, Goldacre, 2012); and, most importantly, pointing out that, on recent evidence, the idea that psychoactive drugs 'treat' specific medical conditions is something that can no longer be sustained (for example, Moncrieff, 2009; Moncrieff *et al.*, 2005). All this has led to a state of crisis in psychiatry. Some psychiatrists (for example, Craddock *et al.*, 2008) see the future of the profession as becoming even more 'scientific' than it is, looking to neuroscience for stabilizing the illness model for mental health, hoping that the Kraepelian illnesses would at last be given credibility by research establishing (it is hoped) the nature of mental illness as diseases of structural change in the brain. An opposing view is expressed in a special article in the *British Journal of Psychiatry*, which postulates a future for psychiatry as a discipline that allies itself with people in trouble (users of mental health services) bringing a necessary medical dimension to a holistic understanding of human problems (Bracken *et al.*, 2012). Both views (in my opinion) tend to ignore the vast array of knowledge about the human condition that exists in the diverse cultural traditions that I have reviewed briefly in this book (Chapter 2), although clearly the latter viewpoint leaves room for psychiatry developing into a system that provides a flexibility that could allow diversity of cultural forms to inform psychiatry (Chapter 11).

Conclusions

The practice of psychiatry and the organization of mental health services in the West (Europe and North America) have undergone quite big changes following the end of WWII. Almost mimicking the great confinement that dominated Europe and America of the eighteenth and nineteenth centuries (when the asylum movement arose), the decades between 1960 and 1990 saw the emergence of a drug-based psychiatry— drugs being the main line of treatments on the assumption that mental illness is caused by chemical imbalance in the brain. This approach is backed by domination of (medical) diagnosis as the main way of conceptualizing problems deemed 'mental' and the imperative towards EBM promoting even further the dependence of bio-medical psychiatry on pharmaceutical agents. Critiques of the drug culture of psychiatry come mainly from sociopolitical (including the transcultural) domains and from psychologists but, more recently, increasingly from psychiatrists and other medical people. In my view, current Euro-American psychiatry lacks credibility as a scientific endeavour and may well be damaging to the social fabric of society, not to speak of the personal damage being suffered by individuals taking some of the drugs prescribed by psychiatrists. That is not to say that some of the drugs used by psychiatrists may not provide some benefit for some people under intense stress or suffering distress—but they only do so if used in small doses for very short periods, mostly as short-term tranquillizers and not as therapy for 'illness'.

Looking back on what happened in the 1970s and 1980s, it would seem that psychiatry was sold to the general public as providing remedies for a variety of personal and social suffering, as well as for madness and later for promoting general well-being. In doing so, it became inextricably linked to the business of producing and marketing potentially powerful drugs. In the asylum days and immediately post-asylum, psychiatrists were pseudo-medical practitioners, the gatekeepers of systems for social exclusion of people unwanted for one reason or another in wider society. As individuals, most professionals working in the asylums at best tried to be supportive towards people they viewed as their responsibility ('patients'); and at worst they maltreated or at least prevented people struggling with human problems from finding their own ways of coping (their own 'salvation', perhaps for misdemeanours and mistakes) by using the power they (especially the psychiatrists) had through positions they held as doctors who were supposed to know about the mind, about behaviour and about 'mental illness'; and clinical psychologists joined in this to a limited extent. But times have changed.

7
Ethnic Problems in the West and Neo-Imperialism Abroad

The 1960s marked a turning point in interactions between the West and the countries of Asia and Africa. Independence movements in Asian and African colonies, which began just before the Second World War (WWII), moved fast following its inglorious termination with the nuclear bombing of two Asian cities, Hiroshima and Nagasaki, in August 1945. The winds of change blew the colonial powers back to their own territories, but still with a big stake in the world outside. The regions that had been colonized and affected by western imperialism in one way or another emerged as countries politically equivalent to those in Europe and North America, but disempowered and underdeveloped economically and politically.

With the end of WWII, European nations looked to ex-colonies for labour to restart their economies and develop transport and health infrastructures. The 1950s to the 1970s saw migration of people from Asia and Africa to western Europe, the UK being particularly popular. For the developing world, this sometimes meant the loss of professionals (the 'brain drain'), often educated at the expense of the state; and hence an overall transfer of resources. For the West, for example, the UK, the migration from Asia and Africa supported the growing economy and health-care systems but created political problems due to resentment of local people at seeing (as it were) the Empire coming home with black people claiming citizenship in the UK. The experiences of slavery and colonialism were repeated in oppression and ghettoization in the emergence of what Hall *et al.* (1978) called 'internal colonies' (p. 351). Indian historian Gyan Prakash (1990) is quoted by Bhabha (1994): 'The Third World, far from being confined to its assigned space, has penetrated the inner sanctum of the "First World" in the process of being "Third Worlded"—arousing, inciting, and affiliating with the subordinated others in the First World...to connect with minority voices' (1990, p. 403). But the postcolonial Third World was powerless to help their Diasporas in Europe.

A general view emerged that the parts of the world that had suffered from industrial and economic underdevelopment during colonial times (see Chapters 4 and 5) would now proceed to 'catch up'. At first it was not easy for the newly independent ex-colonies because of reluctance of the (already) developed rich world to share know-how on manufacturing, but the advent of the 'cold war' provided some windows of opportunity. As the Cold War took hold between the Soviet Union combined with adjoining countries in the 'Eastern Bloc' pitted against the West, the two blocs competed for influence in the 'developing world', now seen as outside both blocs and therefore called the 'Third World'. The West and, to a lesser extent the Soviet Union, provided help to the Third World through aid packages and know-how for economic development as well as armaments. And the World Health Organization (WHO), set up by the United Nations (UN) that had been formed soon after the end of WWII, saw its role as helping the Third World to develop health services.

The chapter begins by focusing on pressures in the first world resulting from migration to Europe from Asia and Africa (a reversal of the nineteenth century migration and also very different in style), resulting in struggles in the UK against racism in psychiatry. The USA, which prided itself on being a 'melting pot' of cultures, began to recognize that racism was rife—James Baldwin spoke of *The Fire Next Time* (1969, book title). Even after the civil rights movement of the 1960s, the country remained as *Two Nations Black and White, Separate, Hostile, and Unequal* (Hacker, 1992, book title) but the extent to which racism influenced psychiatric practice was not explored in the way it was in the UK. Then the chapter examines how psychiatric research in Asia and Africa panned out in the 1960s and 1970s, noting in some detail the first attempt by WHO to take a global view of 'mental health' via a research project called the International Pilot Study of Schizophrenia (IPSS).

Drawing largely on my own observations and using Sri Lanka as an example (because that is the region in Asia I know best), the chapter traces the way western imperialism—this time less overt than it was during colonialism—transferred the cultural products of psychiatry and psychology, by a process of infiltration as the diagnostic model for 'mental health' worked its way into Asia and Africa. During the 30 years from 1980, various terms have been used to describe the apparent dichotomy of the world into two contrasting groups of nations: Developing versus developed, low- and middle-income countries (LMICs) versus high-income countries (HICs); and the Global South as opposed to the Global North. A concluding paragraph summarizes the way the mental health scene has changed in both the West and the Third World.

Problems of racism and the illness model of psychiatry

In the 1970s and 1980s, immigrants to the UK from the Third World faced serious problems of racist hostility and social exclusion. In the mental health field, high levels at which 'schizophrenia' was being diagnosed among black people became a major issue, evoking allegations of racism in psychiatry. A diagnosis given almost exclusively to black people in the 1970s into the 1980s was cannabis psychosis (McGovern and Cope, 1987) reflecting public images, fostered by the media and police, associating race with drug abuse and the attribution of the anger of black youth to their use of cannabis (discussed in Fernando, 2002); later on this diagnosis diminished in use, apparently absorbed into a general 'schizophrenia' or 'psychosis' label. It was evident that diagnoses were linked to specific groups of people seen in racial terms, and that the way diagnoses were made was in effect racist (see Fernando, 2003).

The research field too was not immune from what was soon identified as 'institutional racism' (Fernando, 2003, p. 211). The background is worth considering: In earlier years Kraepelin (1913) had observed that Asian people did not get depressed in the way that Europeans did and, throughout the twentieth century, 'observations' surfaced that Africans and African-Americans did not suffer depression (Green, 1914; Carothers, 1953)—'findings' that were attributed to 'underdevelopment' of non-Europeans (Kraepelin, 1921). These themes were part and parcel of general racist notions in Europe at the time but surprisingly, similar themes emerged in the UK in the 1970s. Julian Leff (1973, 1977, 1986), an eminent researcher at the time based at the Institute of Psychiatry (IOP) in London, developed the idea that people in developing countries, compared to people in the West, had a lower rate of differentiating anxiety symptoms from depressive symptoms except that African-Americans resembled people in the developing world in this respect. He concluded that there was 'a progressive differentiation of the vocabulary of emotion' (Leff, 1986, p. 33) that was an 'evolutionary process' (Leff, 1977, p. 323), which is one of cultural development. A similar way of thinking was voiced by another researcher from the IOP: While referring to non-western cultures as 'primitive cultures' (meaning underdeveloped cultures), Bebbington (1978) argued for 'a provisional syndromal definition of depression as used by a consensus of Western psychiatrists against which cross-cultural anomalies can be tested' (p. 303); in other words, the 'depression' of non-western peoples was hailed as an 'anomaly' not a real illness. All this was included in the body of what was presented (and accepted) as research findings.

Although the main problem in the psychiatric system in the UK was attributed to institutional racism, many of the problems represented cultural insensitivity in the illness model of western psychiatry and the way diagnoses were arrived in psychiatry using a western illness model (for detailed discussions, see Bhui, 2002; Bhui and Olajide, 1999; Fernando, 1988, 1991, 2003; Littlewood and Lipsedge, 1982; Ndegwa and Olajide, 2003; Rack, 1982). Although most of the work exploring these issues were conducted and written up in the UK, the issues were probably pervasive in all European countries where racial and cultural minorities existed.

In the USA, racial differences in diagnostic patterns were noted but not explored very much. An early study in New York (Simon *et al.*, 1973) concluded that 'the diagnostic differences found between blacks and whites were a reflection of US hospital psychiatrists' diagnostic habits [with regard to black people] as much as anything else' (1973, p. 511); and Allon (1971) suggested that stereotyping of black people as genetically inferior may play a part in diagnostic discrepancies. Earlier, Bromberg and Simon (1968) had wondered whether the over-diagnosis of schizophrenia in African-Americans may represent (what they called) 'protest psychosis' (p. 155), essentially an expression of anger by black Americans repudiating white social structures. Much later, this theme was given validity by Jonathan Metzl (2009) in a study of changes in diagnostic pattern at Ionia State Hospital in Michigan from the 1940s onwards until it closed as a mental institution (to become a prison) in the 1970s: Until the early 1960s, schizophrenia was largely 'an illness that afflicted nonviolent, white petty criminals including...women from rural Michigan' but in the mid-1970s, 'schizophrenia was a diagnosis disproportionately applied to...[mainly] African American men from urban Detroit' (2009, pp. xv–xvi). So far, there has been very little study in academia (in the USA) of the ways in which the psychiatric system impacts on African-Americans today. But to judge from Metzl's work, the indication is that the US mental health system is complicit (to say the least) in controlling African-Americans, partially at least through the excessive use of the schizophrenia diagnosis.

However problematic psychiatry was for Britain's black and minority ethnic people and for African-Americans, quite significant changes for the better came about in mental health services on both sides of the Atlantic during the 1970s and 1980s. This was the era when asylums were replaced by community care (Chapter 6). As psychiatry disentangled itself (with some difficulty) from opprobrium of the discredited asylum movement, its image became more acceptable generally, not least in the ex-colonial countries that had suffered from having asylums imposed on them; and, as the medication era seemed (at least in the 1970s) to offer for the first time 'scientific', medical cures for mental illness in a lead up to current bio-medical psychiatry (Chapter 3), its prestige was relatively high in public perceptions. What is striking today is that the inequalities experienced by some racial and cultural minorities continue almost unabated, attributed to a mixture of institutional racism and cultural insensitivity.

While multiculturalism evoked racism in Europe, the presence there of people from Asia, Africa and the Caribbean stimulated an interest of the professional classes in the countries they (the immigrants) came from. Ease of travel and communication together with many books on cultural studies promoted interest in the exotic—as Asia and Africa was to most European people even in the 1980s. Some aspects of Indian and Chinese medicine such as yoga, acupuncture and meditation, began to be talked about and people sought their sources in India and China. It was at that time (the 1980s and the 1990s) that concern about racism in psychiatric practice in the UK reached a peak (Fernando, 2003); and I noticed that one defence by local professionals was to point the finger at Asian and African professionals expressing the concern with comments about what was going on in 'your countries'. Some western-educated British professionals of Asian and African descent (of which there were many) began trying to 'educate' their colleagues in Asia and Africa into upgrading psychiatric services 'back home', telling them how much 'better' it was in the UK; and other British professionals became interested likewise in travelling to these interesting parts of the world as 'experts'. So an insidious process of 'improving' psychiatry in developing countries gradually took off, supported by WHO and non-governmental organizations (NGOs) funded in the West. The experts from the West essentially spread the diagnostic approach for promoting [*sic*] 'mental health', for, after all, this is what they were trained in. But there were other bigger forces at work in spreading psychiatry in the Third World.

Psychiatry penetrating the Global South

Higginbotham and Marsella (1988) analysed the bigger picture within international medical education in the 1970s and 1980s that promoted the expansion of western psychiatry in Southeast Asia. They suggested that western psychiatry was encouraged by some ex-colonial governments as a 'potential tool...for motivating people to embrace the modernization process...[and a means for] coping with individual stress' (p. 553). But they also suggested that the expansion of western psychiatry worked through less direct processes. Asian professionals who had acquired postgraduate education in the West (as a part of obtaining further education in medicine) formed an elite cadre of specialists who assumed positions of influence when they returned to work in their countries of origin; and then, with their connections in the West, international pathways of co-operation were created and centres for training were established locally in ex-colonial countries but always with strong links with Western centres. Thus, whatever systems of diagnoses, treatments and so on that were popular in the West, especially in the UK and the USA, were exported as 'correct' without any input of knowledge on the need to take on board cultural diversity across the world in understanding mental health and illness and the importance of social factors in thinking about these matters, although these issues were in fact being explored by anthropologists and psychiatrists interested in transcultural and cultural studies of mental health and illness (discussed in Chapter 2).

I recall meeting a British child psychiatrist who had never been abroad before who was about to go to India to 'teach' family therapy in the mid-1970s; not only did she not have any knowledge about family life in India, she did not also see any need to acquire any before going. For her and for many others, psychiatry was a technical matter of applying systems of diagnosis and treatment—and teaching in underdeveloped countries was about instructing people on the use of the narrow biomedical models for human problems. I met several other psychiatric specialists in similar positions and I know that they were generally welcomed in countries that had been colonized as people bringing the latest know-how in best practice. The problem was essentially a carry-over of the 'colonial condition' (Bhabha, 1994, pp. 41–42), described in Chapter 5. As a legacy of colonialism, Western arrogance promotes the idea that mental health systems developed in the West and its Euro-American psychiatry are globally applicable, which plays into the impression, sometimes held against common sense by some people in authority in the Third World countries, that development always means westernization. Clearly, looking to the West predominantly rather than to local knowledge may well be beneficial in some fields (such as manufacturing and even medical and surgical techniques) but certainly not appropriate or helpful in mental health development. Thus in the 1970s and 1980s, the modern era of psychiatric imperialism arrived—to last into the present (2013).

Colonialism had imposed the asylum model for mental health services in Asia and Africa but colonial psychiatry was confined to asylums that were few and far between; and psychiatry itself failed to connect with the needs of people in colonized countries of Asia and Africa (Chapter 5). On the whole, ordinary people in the colonies followed their own ways of dealing with (what psychiatry terms) mental illness— possibly no less effectively as the West did at the time. The asylum model was abandoned in the West in the 1970s but, just as the asylum era passed, the great medication revolution took hold in the West (Chapter 6). In the 1960s (after de-colonization), looking from the West, very little was known about mental health needs and practices in the developing world, and so studies appeared to try and fill this gap. Unfortunately, these studies, such as those by Dube (1970) and Elnagar *et al.* (1971) in India, used screening for psychiatric symptoms (that may not have any meaning in the cultural setting concerned) to identify people as 'mentally ill' diagnosed according to psychiatric criteria. Sometimes some studies (for example, that by Murphy and Raman, 1971, in the Mauritius) showed that the outcomes for people deemed to have chronic mental illness seemed to be much better than they were in the UK. But these studies, like others, assumed (incorrectly) that symptoms that seemed to have face validity in the West and diagnoses using the illness model of (western) psychiatry (see Chapter 2) were universally valid. In fact, this and other problems of cross-cultural research (see Chapter 4) were largely unrecognized within health circles at the time.

Although anthropological work during colonial times, albeit done from a western cultural perspective, had indicated that there were vast differences in the ways in which mental health and illness were perceived in non-western as opposed to western societies (Chapter 2) these all failed to impinge on health studies (including those about mental health), mainly because the two disciplines anthropology and psychiatry used very different languages and they hardly talked to each other and transcultural psychiatry, which tried to link the two, had little influence. However, some post-war researchers did appreciate some of the issues involved in cross-cultural understanding in the field of mental health and illness and some tried to get round some of the problems of cross-cultural research.

In the early 1960s, a team from the USA collaborated with a local (western-trained) psychiatrist Adeoye Lambo to study 'psychiatric disorder' among the Yoruba of Aro in western Nigeria (Leighton *et al.*, 1963). Although the study did not eliminate the basic problem of category fallacy (referred to in Chapter 4 and first described by Kleinman, 1977), the Aro study was a significant advance towards understanding the nature of what may have been going on in the mental health field in Africa. But two eminent researchers, Carstairs and Kapur (1976), got much further in southern India with a study in the village of Kota in Karnataka state (referred to in Chapter 4). These researchers collaborated with local people to devise research instruments to measure emotional problems as seen by people of the area of study (in southern India) and tested them out in pilot studies. Initially, the researchers spent some time in exploring the relationship between what could be identified as 'symptoms' and people's 'need' (for help) as evidenced by their consulting indigenous healers, declaring inability to cope with everyday tasks or social relations, or decline in day to day functioning. Using the 'symptoms' that seemed valid (as 'illness') for the particular population, the researchers compared three groups in the village that seemed to be naturally seen as distinctive from each other. The findings indicated higher than expected rates of what may add up to 'neuroses' with marked differences in rates between caste groups. They drew the conclusion that personal suffering presented with symptoms that were peculiar to each sociocultural setting and suggested that by identifying 'cases' by such a bottom-up way, services can be built up consisting of a plurality of interventions acceptable to people concerned.

It is noteworthy that the Kota study obtained most of its subjects (for deriving their findings on 'need') from among clients of indigenous healers. It is then safe to assume that many of the people who were ultimately identified as suffering 'neuroses' would have been attending such healers. In the area that the research was based, the 'professional healers', some practising Ayurveda (an Indian medical system), were distinct from priests and holy men who exercised their healing powers through supernatural means; the former had 'undergone a period of training to achieve their expertise and charged a fee for their services' (1976, p. 58). Many people with a self-perceived 'need' had consulted both traditional healers and western (allopathic) doctors: 'The contradictory "causal" terminology used by doctors and the traditional healers apparently presented no problem to a Kota villager. "There are many ways to truth" claimed a university educated Brahmin, echoing the core philosophy of Hinduism, which effortlessly embraces contradictions' (1976, p. 66.). Indeed, this acceptance of a plurality of explanations and (in the case of illness) treatment modalities characterizes most Asian cultures.

Perhaps Morris Carstairs and Ravi Kapur were unique individuals able to straddle two widely different cultures—far ahead of their times in that respect. I remember a newspaper report on a visit to Sri Lanka (then called Ceylon) by Morris Carstairs in the early 1950s. On being asked about his impressions of services for mental illness, he declined to comment on the asylum near Colombo but spoke highly of the services at the Buddhist temple that I knew (mentioned in Chapter 4) Many years later (in the 1970s) I was to meet Morris Carstairs in Edinburgh when he helped to form a transcultural psychiatry movement in Scotland that later developed into the Transcultural Psychiatry Society (UK) that lobbied for anti-racist action in psychiatry throughout the 1980s (Chapter 6). Ravi Kapur went on to head up the National Institute for Mental Health at Bangalore which was at the time a centre for social psychiatry, although I believe it is no longer so having espoused a mainly bio-medical approach derived from Euro-American practice. The new model for research with an East–West collaboration pioneered by Carstairs and Kapur way back in the 1970s attracted some attention but was not promoted by the power brokers of psychiatry and the scene was rather dramatically changed when WHO, informed by the very traditional (British) IOP, set about getting some basic facts (or so they thought) by carrying out a survey called the IPSS (WHO, 1973, 1975, 1979) using western diagnoses (see the following section).

Unexpected results of WHO studies

Having identified cohorts of people diagnosed with 'schizophrenia', the IPSS carried out assessments at two to five year follow-up studies (Sartorius *et al.*, 1986; WHO, 1973) and then at 13–17-year follow-up studies (Hopper and Wanderling, 2000; Sartorius *et al.*, 1996). Unexpectedly and possibly to the surprise of the researchers, outcomes for people seen as seriously mentally ill (albeit in psychiatric terms) were actually *better* in non-western settings. People diagnosed as suffering from 'schizophrenia' in non-western settings (India and Nigeria, for example) had better outcomes than those of people in western settings (in the UK and the USA, for example) both in terms of symptom relief and social recovery. The IPSS was described briefly in Chapter 4 as being flawed as a transcultural research strategy because it ignored category fallacy (described in Chapter 4). The approach in IPSS was the traditional epidemiological one of defining an illness (in terms of Kraepelinian nosology) and measuring it at various stages of (what is called) its natural history, disregarding category fallacy (described in Chapter 4). The basic instrument used for evaluating patients was the Present State Examination (PSE) (Wing *et al.*, 1974) which had been described by its founder as 'a standardised form of the psychiatric diagnostic interview ordinarily used in Western Europe' (Wing, 1978, p. 103). It would seem that the research method was both culturally insensitive and somewhat patronizing. However, the outcome studies suggested that the therapeutic context for recovery may have been better in non-western settings for some reason; indeed there were articles on why this may have been so (for example, by Cooper and Sartorius, 1977; Halliburton, 2004; Hopper, 1991; Leff *et al.*, 1990; Warner, 1985), but no attempt by WHO was made to follow up this lead by perhaps questioning seriously the validity of psychiatric diagnosis or at least examining how non-western sociocultural environments may be conducive to good outcomes for 'illness'. It would seem that the underlying assumption of WHO researchers was that 'illness' had to be treated and that non-western societies could not possibly be better than western ones. In any case, the significance of IPSS findings had very little impact on the bio-medical revolution (search for better and better drugs) that was taking off at that time in the West (Chapter 6).

The main result of IPSS was to establish that a reliable method of diagnosing schizophrenia in terms already established in the West is possible, so long as people using the concept are carefully trained in its use. In other words, a diagnosis can be applied reliably to a group of people presenting at (western-type) medical institutions in various countries, once the diagnosticians were trained to use the same, or similar, criteria for making the diagnosis. The hospital centres used for the IPSS were considered to be 'centres of excellence' because they were applying western models of diagnosis and treatment. This approach to psychiatric diagnosis could be likened to the diagnosis of sin: Such a diagnosis can be highly reliable across cultures and ethical barriers if people making the diagnosis (say Roman Catholic priests) are trained to adhere to a particular system.

Apart from its negative effects of being misleading and unscientific, I believe that the IPSS had significant insidious social effects by inducing cultural shifts that caused some degree of 'forced globalization' (as described in Chapter 1): The prestige that the PSE obtained as a result of its use in such a major international study as IPSS gave it undeserved credibility as a tool in measuring mental illness across cultures. Although never validated properly anywhere in the world, by the 1980s, the use of the PSE had spread around the globe through training provided directly or indirectly by prestigious institutes in London; and it was used in various settings—for example, in Africa (Orley and Wing, 1979), Egypt (Okasha and Ashour, 1981) and South Africa (Swartz *et al.*, 1985). It became the gold standard for diagnosing 'schizophrenia'. In the global scene, the PSE and indeed the diagnosis of schizophrenia which was seriously being criticized in the 1960s became integrated in the 1980s into sociopolitical systems of the Third World. The ex-colonies were being colonized all over again—this time by psychiatry.

Like the IPSS, later studies conducted by WHO, the Collaborative Study on the Assessment and Reduction of Psychiatric Disability (Jablensky *et al.*, 1980) and the Determinants of Outcome of Severe Mental Disorders (Sartorius *et al.*, 1986; WHO, 1986), took as their starting point assumptions about the universal validity of western diagnostic formulations. The latter (the most recent of the WHO studies) used subjects drawn from people making contact with both western-type psychiatric facilities as well as indigenous healers, religious shrines and other sources of help (Sartorius *et al.*, 1986), thereby gathering under an umbrella of bio-medical 'mental illness' a variety of human experiences that may be related to social functioning, spiritual life or whatever—and should have remained so especially in non-western cultural settings. All through the series of WHO studies in the 1970s, there was an assumption that, if a system that is developed in Europe and seemingly suitable for western cultures (although that too is now being questioned—Chapter 6) it is good enough for everyone.

1970s Onwards

As diagnostic systems were formalized and tightened up in the post-war period, psychiatry began to look more like a medical discipline that was able to diagnose reliably specific illnesses and even claim possible cures (Chapter 6). Also, the revulsion against locking people up merely for being different, together with the advent of powerful drugs that could suppress overt 'disturbed' behaviour was resulting in opening up of the asylums and a general call for de-institutionalization. The asylum approaches during colonialism had not cut much ice in Asia and Africa with the common people. And even during the immediate post-war period, the asylums in Asia and Africa remained anomalies of the colonial era—institutions representing alien views established by outsiders who did not know better and did not understand local people.

In spite of their poor experience of psychiatry in colonial times, the ex-colonial developing nations were gradually enticed into the psychiatric fold in the 1970s. 'Science' was seen as the way forward in all fields; and psychiatry was presented as a medical system that was as scientific as other branches of medicine, many of which were dealing effectively with serious illnesses of various sorts. In the UK, a Royal College of Psychiatrists was recognized as being of equivalent status to other medical royal colleges.

In the Third World, psychiatry gradually lost some of its colonial taint and assumed an aura of respectability. And the obvious advances of technological medicine in treating successfully many diseases rubbed off onto psychiatry seemingly recognized by then (in the West) as a branch of medicine. In this context, and encouraged by some western-trained professionals returning to their own countries, people in developing countries looked to scientific medicine and its (apparent) counterpart psychiatry for progress in health care; and the idea of 'mental illness' and even of 'mental health' gradually took hold in some circles. In other words, psychiatry, riding on the back of scientific medicine, was taken up at the expense of neglecting indigenous systems for 'mental health' (still seen by most people in spiritual and social terms) that had apparently served them well until then but needed developing, updating and regulating. The prestige of the IPSS gave credibility to the 'schizophrenia' diagnosis and added to the imperial message that psychiatric illness was a superior model to whatever else was being followed.

When I went back to Sri Lanka after qualifying in medicine and applied to work at the asylum near Colombo in 1960, my relatives were puzzled that I should expect to practise 'medicine' in an asylum. There was little conception among the general public of people who were locked away there being 'ill' in any way. The concept of the 'mind' getting 'ill' was a strange one—the concept was not embedded in the culture (Chapters 2 and 4). In fact, I had difficulty in finding the asylum at first because I persisted in asking the way to a hospital, until someone suddenly realized that I wanted the *pissan kotuwa* (Sinhala for 'stockade for lunatics'). However, by the mid-1980s, the mental hospital was seen as a medical institute and ordinary people were talking about 'schizophrenia'; and physicians wanted to know about the latest drugs for depression and anxiety that local people were experiencing as a result of political violence and economic instability that was spreading in the country. By the early 1990s, nearly all the people locked up in the asylum were thought to be schizophrenics (personal observation). Where colonial psychiatry had failed, postcolonial imperialism (epitomized by the IPSS) was succeeding to infiltrate minds of ordinary people by playing into the allure of apparent 'scientific progress'.

In the 1980s and 1990s, social and political issues that had been left unresolved during the colonial era—or sometimes worsened by 'divide-and-rule' policies during colonial rule—were bearing their bitter fruit in the shape of rivalries and inter-group conflicts in Asia and Africa. Ethnic antagonisms coupled with easy availability of weapons led to vicious civil wars in some ex-colonial countries. On my visits to Sri Lanka, I noticed with dismay the rise of a local brand of racism promoted by political forces and fanned by outside interests promoting instability, erupting into armed conflict. As in many other similar situations, western NGOs descended on the country, usually with an overt 'humanitarian' remit, offering practical help but, in the field of 'mental health development', spreading psychiatric models for human suffering in the process. For example, western-trained therapists taught 'trauma therapy', advocated use of 'anti-psychotics' for people going through spiritual crises or counselled people who were depressed on how they should change their ways of thinking about themselves, advising against religious and other indigenous ways that local people had for dealing with social suffering and personal problems. However, admittedly many individuals working in NGOs were well-intentioned and seemed oblivious of the harm they were doing, and indeed some of the practical work they did was helpful in the circumstances. The problem was a matter of the unintended harm that came with the intended benefits.

Towards the turn of the century, humanitarian organizations multiplied rapidly focusing entirely on the Third World, arriving whenever there was any suffering as a result of disasters or conflicts. The ex-colonial powers, responsible for some of the worst human rights violations before and during WWII, were now espousing a 'mission' to carry out humanitarian activity all over the world, intervening politically and sometimes militarily in order to do so. The era of western intervention became reminiscent of nineteenth-century colonization to 'civilize' the natives. Humanitarian work in the field of mental health focused on the western model of trauma-therapy, a booming psychiatric industry as a result of the invention of 'post-traumatic stress disorder' in the USA during the post-Vietnam upheaval (Young, 1995), but soon involved spreading diagnosis-medication-based bio-medical psychiatry (see Watters, 2011).

In Sri Lanka (which I use as an example of the sort of changes that were taking place all over the Third World) during the 1990s into the first decade of the twenty-first century, there were many NGOs staffed by well-meaning but misguided professionals carrying out mental health projects derived from traditional psychiatric theories and using psychiatric language. And with psychological therapies for trauma came medications for relieving depression that 'traumatized' people were diagnosed as suffering from. During and after the civil war and the disaster caused by the 2004 tsunami in Sri Lanka, people in areas affected by conflict and disaster were enticed by resource-rich NGOs to opt for 'scientific' psychiatric and psychological treatment in preference to their (allegedly) 'superstitious' beliefs and their cultural support networks, religious systems and so on—just as 200 years earlier their predecessors had been persuaded by Christian missionaries to worship a modern all-powerful god from the West.

The subtle but powerful imposition of psychiatry was supported by some western-educated professional elites in the Third World and, invariably, the activities of the pharmaceutical companies. Even as early as the 1970s, tranquillizers and anti-depressants were reaching bazaars in Asia (Carstairs, 1973), and psychotropics were being marketed in most LMICs by the end of 1990s. It is reported that psychotropic drug sales in Pakistan for just one year between July 2003 and June 2004 was worth Rs. 2.76 billion (US$46.77 million) (Khan, 2006). Correspondingly, since the early 1980s, diagnosis-based psychiatry that feeds the marketing of psychotropics has been adopted in most western-style asylums that have been renamed 'hospitals' and even in psychiatric clinics in the community that have come on the scene (see Jain and Jadhav, 2009). However, in many non-western regions of the world, ways of thinking of most ordinary people are inconsistent with models of illness and health that underpin psychiatry (Chapters 2 and 3); and even now (2013) they generally prefer to access indigenous ways of managing problems that amount in psychiatric language to mental illness, although increasingly the psychiatric language is being adopted by social and professional elites in these regions. Also, indigenous therapies are being pushed out by economic forces and the marketing of diagnosis (see Chapter 8).

Conclusions

As migrants from ex-colonies in Asia, Africa and the Caribbean settled in the UK and other European countries during the 1980s and

1990s, 'ethnic issues' in mental health services and psychiatry became evident reflecting the general problems of racism in western societies and the likelihood that racism, coupled with an insensitivity to cultural diversity, was integrated into the psychiatric diagnostic system. Abroad, that is in the very ex-colonial countries that migrants had come from, western ideologies, including those inherent in psychiatry and psychology, permeated via activities of NGOs funded by western agencies, (western) 'experts' sent to 'advise' and the work of a rising professional elite within the countries themselves often eager to imitate the West. All this is reminiscent of what missionaries and colonial civil servants (many of whom were from the colonies themselves but educated into western ways of thinking) did in earlier times. So home-grown racism in the UK was paralleled by imperialism abroad.

A UK report generally called the Orville Blackwood Report (SHSA, 1993) pointed to racism in mental health services as 'subtle' rather than 'overt'. Other reports on racism in the police force (Home Department, 1999) pointed to its 'institutional', rather than personal, nature. In similar vein, racism involved in over-diagnosis of schizophrenia in African-Americans in the USA has been called 'institutionalized racism' (Metzl, 2009, p. 146). From the 1990s onwards, institutional or subtle racism in the Global North appears to be matched by similar process of indirect imperialism, sometimes with a racist edge to it, instituted through economic pressures imposing cultural change in the Global South. But oppressions are not just black and white; the clash is not so much between the North and South but, as Navarro (2007) points out (in a slightly different context), between the *dominant* classes in the North and South as opposed to *dominated* classes—the poor, the disposed, the socially excluded in both regions. In this context, the post-asylum image of psychiatry in the North as a medical science that carries scientific cures (unlike the asylum psychiatry of colonial times)

Table 7.1 1970s onwards: North and South

Global North	Global South
Subtle racism (ethnic issues)	Indirect imperialism
Institutional racism	Cultural change
Psychiatry as medical science	Penetration of psychiatry
Post-asylum	'Scientific', 'evidence based'

has enabled bio-medical psychiatry to penetrate the South as supposedly scientific and evidence based (Table 7.1).

Chapter 8 considers how the spread of psychiatry in the Global South is being maintained through political and economic forces in spite of serious discontents (with psychiatry) in the Global North and what can be done to remedy this state of affairs.

8
International Politics of Mental Health and Psychiatry

Health, it is sometimes said, is political because 'like any other resource or commodity under a neo-liberal economic system, some social groups have more of it than others... its social determinants are amenable to political interventions... [and]... power is exercised over it as part of a wider economic, social and political system' (Bambra *et al.*, 2005, p. 187). The political nature of health is nowhere more evident than in the case of mental health since the very concept 'mental health' is somewhat removed from other aspects of 'health'; it lacks objective criteria for identifying deviation from health into 'illness' rendering psychiatric diagnoses scientifically invalid and of doubtful utility (Chapter 6); and it is strongly dependent on how 'mind' is understood, what 'mental' actually *means*, and the variation of this meaning across cultural traditions (Chapter 2). In fact, it would seem that the promotion of 'mental health' in many societies would be better served if discourse focuses primarily on its social, psychological and spiritual ingredients, rather than (as if often the case) its medical dimension. Recent focus at the World Health Organization (WHO) on 'social determinants of health' (see below) seems a very positive sign because follow through on addressing the problems in the social dimension of health worldwide should have far reaching improvements in social conditions and well-being all round and greater sense of fulfilment for people, both as individuals and communities.

This chapter begins by discussing the sociopolitical context of mental health and psychiatry. This is a continuing story that may well change radically if lessons from the current (2008 onwards) economic setback to western capitalism results in a shift away from neo-liberalism and regulation and control for the public good of big business, including the pharmaceutical companies, although there is little indication so far that will happen very soon. Then, the chapter looks more specifically at the global politics of the world of psychiatry and mental health—although clearly 'mental health' may well be a misnomer for the vast array of issues around well-being, community cohesion, personal happiness and all the rest that it covers. The chapter includes a section on a movement to spread psychiatry worldwide supported by the National Institute for Mental Health in the USA (or NIMH-USA), the WHO, and seemingly pharmaceutical companies. Finally the chapter draws some conclusions about the present state of play in the international scene in the field of mental health, with special reference to low- and middle-income countries (LMICs).

Sociopolitical context of health and illness

The past three decades have seen geopolitical changes that affect the world heath scene significantly. Neo-liberal ideologies, implemented through political and economic policies, began in the 1980s, sometimes called the 'Thatcher–Reagan years', and spread to many parts of the western world and even to developing countries. Neo-liberalism advocates, and to some extent implements, economic liberalization, de-regulation of big business (including the banks and pharmaceutical companies), open markets (with so-called 'free trade' that often contains in-built protection of western interests), privatization of state assets and promotion of the private sector in all fields, *including health*. Although neo-liberal policies were supposed to improve living standards all round through a trickle down of wealth, this has clearly not often happened. Vincente Navarro (2009), Professor of Public Policy, Sociology and Policy Studies at the John Hopkins (USA), points out that health inequalities have actually increased as a result of neo-liberalism both in the developing countries and the USA.

Neo-liberalism did not spread globally untouched by other processes. In the 1980s, 'Reagonomics' and 'Thatcherism', the political arm of neo-liberalism, 'attached to a nationalistic imagery that, from time to time, exploded into hyper-patriotism, saw themselves as the torch-bearers of an Anglo-American civilization anchored in the ideals of political liberty, free-market commerce and love of country' (Steger and Roy, 2010, p. 43). In the Blair-Clinton-Bush era that followed Reagan and Thatcher, US hegemony and the power of US-led big business (supported by UK) was thrust down the throats of most developing nations by a mixture of hard-power (economic, political and military actions) and soft-power (diplomatic and political pressures, economic aid and so on)—for definitions of hard- and soft-power see Steger and Roy (2010). And neo-liberalism, spread worldwide, has been associated with—Navarro (2007) argues *resulted* in—greater incidence of poverty and widening of health inequalities across most parts of the world (Coburn, 2004; Navarro, 1998).

In the second decade of the twenty-first century (the present),

> neo-liberalism is the dominant ideology permeating the public poli-cies of many governments in developed and developing countries and of international agencies such as the World Bank, International Monetary Fund, World Trade Organization and many agencies of the United Nations, including the World Health Organization .... The major beneficiaries of these policies are the dominant classes of both the developed and the developing countries.
>
> (Navarro, 2007, p. 47)

Taking on board the economic advances in several developing coun-tries during the 1980s onwards, Navarro (2007) argues that the primary conflict in the world is now not so much between the rich North and the poor South; it is between the dominant classes of the North and South and the dominated classes of the North and South. In the mental health field, many professional bodies, such as those represent-ing psychiatrists—although not all individual psychiatrists—tend to fall into the former (dominant class). WHO too, at least as far as its policies on mental health are concerned, has been swept into this dominant class stream, possibly because of its dependence for resources on the rich western countries and, it seems increasingly, on private big busi-ness (see below). This is the context in which recent interest in the social determinants of health needs to be considered.

Social determinants of health

The report (CSDH, 2008) produced by a WHO Commission chaired by Michael Marmot pinned the cause of many of the social deter-minants on 'the emergence of a dominant (sometimes referred to as "neo-liberal") orthodoxy in global institutions' (2008a, p. 166). This WHO Commission proposed three types of action: Improving daily liv-ing conditions; tackling inequitable distribution of power, money and resources; and measuring and understanding the problem and assess-ing the impact of action. Navarro (2009) was quick to point out that all these laudable aims if pursued in practice would necessitate an overall re-distribution of wealth, but WHO singularly failed to confront this fact. Action on social determinants of health would entail changes at international and national levels—action that would threaten the power of the rich countries (Mooney, 2012), so the question then is whether these (western) powers will try to block such action; recent experience shows they may well—for example, Navarro (2009) points to US and European Union opposition to Chavez government in Venezuela that tried to implement wealth re-distribution.

The views expressed in Marmot's report (see above) were soon supported by the book *The Spirit Level* by Wilkinson and Picket (2010). The conference at Rio de Janeiro in October 2011, *All for Equity* (WHO, 2011a), reiterated the importance of addressing social determinants of health and spoke of the urgency for action, pointing to the need to 'identify basic principles methods and strategies... strengthen political commitment... and share experiences, challenges and technical knowledge' (2011a, p. 2). But WHO did not come up with plans or strategies for such action—this being left to individual governments. The late Gavin Mooney (2012) wondered 'having identified the problem, why then back off from indicating how to deal with it?' (2012, p. 388). And he argued: '[I]f global health and global inequities in health are to be improved, another form of political economy must be found— one based on community values rather than the individualistic values of neoliberalism' (p. 383). Significantly, in the foreword to *All for Equity*, WHO's Director General, Margaret Chan, stated: 'Globalization was purported to be the rising tide that would lift all boats. However, the reality has been that it lifted the big boats but tended to sink or swamp smaller ones' (WHO 2011a, p. 1). If, as it seems to be the case, WHO is either unable or unwilling to say what needs to be done by governments, private (profit-making) businesses, especially the pharmaceutical industry, may enter the scene and push mental health development in a direction that would certainly not be based on community values. This may be happening already: a consultation set up by WHO in Ontario (Canada) (WHO, 2011b) suggests engagement with the private sector—something an earlier meeting in Australia hosted by the Government of South Australia and WHO (Kickbusch, 2010) had done too. In fact, WHO itself may well be heading this way (see below).

Spreading psychiatry through political pressures

Until the mid-1990s, international health (IH) was the commonly used term to refer to health in countries outside the West including (after the end of the colonial era) ex-colonies. IH focused on 'tropical diseases' referred to health status and needs in developing countries and to comparative analysis of national level health systems. In the mid-1990s, IH became 'global health' for two reasons (McInnes and Lee, 2012): First to provide 'a political boost to long neglected public health problems... [and] ... second to call for a paradigm shift in response to how human health is being affected in new ways by global interconnectedness' (McInnes and Lee, 2012, p. 8). In any case the literature on aspects of global health, such as global health governance, since 1990s represents a major change in the way health is being envisaged internationally. It should be noted at this point that *mental health* is not included within the 'global health' category (see below). The recent introduction of the term 'global mental health' is discussed later in this chapter.

Once WHO was established in 1948 as a part of the post-war arrangement (Chapter 4) there was a slow increase of international health activities in which the ex-colonial Third World was included. In the case of public health, narratives that surfaced tended to focus on national health strategies rather than international cooperation. However, gradually, a broad consensus developed around a need to strengthen collective action to address health concerns across the world. A major development in the approach to health in WHO circles arrived with the Alma-Ata declaration in 1978 at the International Conference on Primary Health Care (WHO, 1978). The first paragraph of the declaration stated that

> health, which is a state of complete physical, mental and social well-being, and not merely the absence of disease or infirmity, is a fundamental human right and that the attainment of the highest possible level of heath is a most important world-wide social goal whose realization requires the action of many other social and economic sectors in addition to the health sector

and then went on to draw attention to the 'existing gross inequality in the health status of the people particularly between developing countries as well as within countries' (WHO, 1988, p. 7). Out of this came the goal of health for all (HFA) and the UN Millennium Summit in 2000 reached a consensus on a set of eight Millennium Development Goals (MDGs) targeted for fulfilment by the year 2015 namely (Hulme, 2007):

1. Eradicate extreme poverty and hunger;
2. Achieve universal primary education;
3. Promote gender equality and empower women;

4. Reduce child mortality;
5. Improve maternal health;
6. Combat HIV/AIDS, malaria, and other diseases;
7. Ensure environmental sustainability; and
8. Develop a global partnership for development (pp. 23–6).

The discourse on MDGs did not include mental health and mental illness for very good reasons (see Chapters 2, 4, 6 and 7). To summarize these: (a) There was no *global* definition of *mental* health, the very concept 'mental health' being largely determined by culture and so variable across the world; (b) there was no clear definition of illness in relation to the 'mind' that applied cross-culturally; and (c) the nosology of 'mental illness' used in western psychiatry was neither scientifically valid nor useful when used across cultures.

It seemed in the 1990s that WHO officials were sympathetic to the viewpoint that in developing mental health services, 'mental health' had to be defined in culturally sensitive ways that suited the cultural traditions and social conditions in different parts of the world (Chapter 2) and moreover that what was seen as 'mental' in western traditions may well be outside the parameters of how 'health' was normally seen in many other cultural traditions. In other words, people at WHO, like many people in transcultural and cultural psychiatry circles, were persuaded that in developing services for mental health in non-western cultural settings, local indigenous meanings in different parts of the world must be taken on board; merely translating western concepts and imposing 'treatment' based on these, were to be avoided. So, for instance, 'mental health' had to be translated as something much wider and more holistic—for example, as 'well-being' (see Chapter 10). Neither, the American DSM (APA, 1994) nor its own ICD (WHO, 1992) was of much use in these circumstances.

A parallel issue around the understanding of 'mental health' arose during emergency humanitarian work carried out by various agencies during the 1980s onwards, particularly in non-western settings. Populations affected by disasters and conflict experienced enormous social suffering at times and workers in humanitarian agencies were impelled to provide what they called 'psychosocial support' which some health sectors tended to call 'mental health care'. Not surprisingly, there was often failure in co-ordination between agencies on the ground. In 1992, the UN General Assembly set up a group of the heads of various UN and non-UN humanitarian organizations to sort this out. This group, the Inter-Agency Standing Committee (IASC, 2007) devised guidelines to promote inter-sector co-ordination based on a composite term 'mental health and psychosocial support' (MHPSS) 'to describe any type of local or outside support that aims to protect or promote psychosocial well-being and/or prevent or treat mental disorder' (2007, p. 1). The report strongly supported by WHO stressed the importance of providing basic services and security first, then community and family support, focussed non-specialized supports and then finally (for a very small number only) specialized psychiatric services.

Policy shifts at WHO

In the 1990s, to judge by WHO publications and statements made by officials of its Department of Mental Health and Substance Abuse (DMHSA), the culturally sensitive view of mental health development (as described above and explored in many of the chapters in this book) was reflected in WHO policies and the views of Benedetto Saraceno who, till early 2000s, was director of DMHSA. But in the early 2000s, there seemed to be uncertainty developing around them: For example, a WHO document in 2004 referred to 'initial difficulty faced by researchers and policy-makers in this [mental health] field... [that are]... related to the similarities and boundaries between the concepts of mental health and mental illness and between prevention and promotion' (WHO, 2004, p. 16); and a foreword by Saraceno (2004) in another document stated: 'One of the crucial issues in the implementation of evidence-based prevention is the real-life applicability of laboratory-proven programmes, especially in widely varying cultural and resource settings. Rigorous controlled effectiveness trials seem to provide more definite evidence but in turn are less amenable to wider application across the world' (p. 3).

WHO documents moved towards a (western) psychiatric bias with talk of interventions based on 'evidence' from Europe and North America using western DSM or ICD categories of illness for identifying 'need' in the developing world. For example, WHO's *Nations for Mental Health* (WHO, 2002) and its more important *World Health Report 2001, Mental Health: New Understanding, New Hope* (WHO, 2001) both drew attention to the 'burden of mental and behavioural disorders' interpreted on the lines of ICD-10 nosology (WHO, 1992) and stressed the importance of diagnosing these 'using clinical methods [of psychiatry] that are similar to those used for physical disorders' (p. 21). A paper by Shekar Saxena *et al.* (2006)—Saxena by then being the Director for the DMHSA at WHO—apparently setting out WHO's official policy for the future, talked of there being 'sufficient evidence indicating the efficacy of interventions...preventing psychiatric symptoms and new cases of mental disorders. [and]...specific interventions to increase resilience'; and then of 'mental disorders and positive mental health....as inter-related components of a single concept of mental health' (p. 5), with no reference to cultural diversity or even to mental health and mental illness being even distantly related to social-political context.

The question arises as to how WHO decision-making actually works. Does it carry out proper systematic reviews and if so why are they not published? How much of WHO policy is driven by political forces and/or lobbying by groups that may have economic interests in promoting par-ticular viewpoints? Oxman *et al.* (2007) of the Norwegian Knowledge Centre for the Health Services carried out an evaluation of WHO pro-cedures for decision-making, including decision-making in the mental health field. They found that 'systematic reviews and concise summaries of findings are rarely used for developing recommendations. Instead, processes usually rely heavily on experts in a particular specialty, rather than representatives of those who will have to live with the recom-mendations or on experts in particular methodological areas' (p. 1883). In such a situation, external exigencies and/or pressures from 'experts' from powerful countries or vested interests could potentially play a part in policy change. One exigency could well be a question of financial support; and reliance on external 'experts' (rather than internal inde-pendent reviews) means being open to agencies or people from rich countries with the means to pay—and on the private sector with its own agendas. Power to influence policy often goes with the ability to pay for implementing it.

The financing of the work of WHO is complicated; the agency depends on both (means tested) contributions from member states as well as voluntary contributions (VCs) from member states, and also on non-government funders such as foundations, investment banks and NGOs (Bussard, 2012). Since the mid-1990s, WHO has looked to VCs for financing much of its work. Science journalist Sonia Shah (2011) wrote in *Foreign Affairs*: 'In 1970, these private contributions constituted a quarter of the agency's budget. By 2008, they constituted nearly 80 per cent. Thus, it is now the private donors, not the WHO, who can call the shots in Geneva, and thereby shape the global health agenda' (p. 3). It seems that a 10–15 per cent drop in contributions from the public sector (for example, member states and international institutions) left WHO 300 million dollar deficit for 2011 (Bussard, 2012). Although the ten million dollars in donations from pharmaceutical companies that it received in the two years 2010–2011 (Harmer, 2012) does not go very far in solving its financial problems, it does mean that WHO may well look to greater support from big business. This may well result in compromising its policies to suit private donors—for example, in support of medication-based programmes as opposed to programmes that promote indigenous non-western therapies.

In 2008, WHO published its *Mental Health Gap Action Programme* (WHO, 2008a) directed at LMICs. Lumping together mental, neurological and substance abuse disorders and prioritizing 'depression, schizophrenia and other psychotic disorders, suicide, epilepsy, dementia disorders due to use of illicit drugs, and mental disorders in children', the report says: 'The essence of the *mhGAP* is partnership to reinforce and to accelerate efforts and increase investment towards providing services to those who do not have any' (pp. 3–4). The talk is of 'evidence-based interventions to address the priority conditions' listed as psychiatric diagnoses and 'intervention packages' for their treatment (p. 11) where medications used in Euro-American psychiatry play the dominant role. The process of 'scaling up' services in LMICs to match those in high-income countries (HICs) seems to mean the imposition of these interventions (mainly medications) by dealing with obstacles to their imposition. In fact, the report talks of establishing new partners and one wonders who these partners may be; the likelihood in such a scenario is that Big Pharma will be one either by directly funding (and hence influencing) mental health service development or by indirect means such as subsidizing training that tends to promote pharmaceutical agents or giving donations to NGOs or even governments to implement programmes that would create markets for their products. (Evidence available in the public domain of support by Big Pharma for global mental health programmes is referred to below.)

Today (in 2013), WHO seems to disregard the problems inherent in applying western models of 'mental illness' worldwide (Chapters 2, 4, 5, 6 and 7) and appears to have reverted to the colonial-type thinking of its discredited International Pilot Study of Schizophrenia (IPSS) (Chapter 7). Yet, WHO publications until the early 2000s had projected a very different message: For example, a publication placed on its website in the 1990s and still (August 2013) there states: 'Mental health refers to a broad array of activities directly or indirectly related to the mental well-being component included in the WHO's definition of health: "A state of complete physical, mental and social well-being, and not merely the absence of disease"' (WHO, 2008b, p. 1). And advice from WHO Regional Office for South-East Asia (2008) which was on its website until mid-2009 and downloaded by me and used in teaching in Sri

Lanka, went even further away from the traditional psychiatric model of mental health by emphasizing the need (in developing countries) to work closely with indigenous systems of healing and medicine. But another definition, this time of 'mental disorders' rather than mental health, has appeared on a WHO website very recently: 'Mental disorders comprise a broad range of problems, with different symptoms. However, they are generally characterized by some combination of abnormal thoughts, emotions, behaviour and relationships with others. Examples are schizophrenia, depression, mental retardation and disorders due to drug abuse. Most of these disorders can be successfully treated' (WHO, 2010, p. 1) and the website has descriptions of various diagnoses drawn from psychiatric nosology.

To summarize, WHO documents that were sensitive to voices from transcultural psychiatry and the information it must have been getting from the (culturally) non-western LMICs—and in my view represented approaches to mental health development that are in line with modern thinking—appear to have been taken off WHO websites in the early 2000s and substituted with documents that support a psychiatric approach, namely one that emphasizes the need to make diagnoses according to western nosology. Such as approach moves away from a public health approach (of 'mental health') sensitive to cultural diversity and towards a psychiatric (medical) one (of 'mental disorders') that is not. Whether this suggests a change of WHO ideology or not, it is certainly a change of direction and shift in WHO policy.

Movement for Global Mental Health (MGMH)

In 2007, *The Lancet* (a prestigious British medical journal) published a series of articles launched by its editor (Horton, 2007) arguing (without providing any convincing evidence) that 'disturbances of mental health' are neglected in LMICs, that 'low-income countries and civil society groups are crying for help'; and that 'there is already a strong evidence base on which to scale up mental health services' world-wide (Horton, 2007, p. 806). The *Lancet* articles defined problems to be tackled in 'mental health' in terms of psychiatric and neurological diagnoses and failed to address the problems inherent in looking to evidence-based medicine (EMB) (discussed in Chapter 6) when considering psychiatric practice—something particularly important in developing mental health services in non-western settings (see later).

In 2010, the joint directors of a newly formed 'Centre for Global Mental Health' based in the UK announced in an article ('commentary') in the *Journal of the American Medical Association* that a 'new global health field comes of age' called 'Global Mental Health' (Patel and Prince, 2010, p. 1976) and that a Movement for Global Mental Health (MGMH) had been formed with its own website. And soon, various supporting systems, such as a training course and conferences and even public lectures appeared on the scene. The point was made by some commentators that the term 'global mental health' lacks credibility—Summerfield (2012) dubbed it an 'oxymoron' (p. 3) because the parameters of *mental health* and *mental illness* cannot be measured in ways that are universally valid, the meaning given to them being determined largely by cultural background and social context (Chapter 2). The choice of the term 'global' qualifying mental health has been taken widely to imply that the meaning of 'mental health' is the same worldwide in all cultural settings and that the same remedies for mental illness are equally applicable worldwide; and when these remedies are referred to as 'evidence-based' (as MGMH does), they clearly refer to treatments used by Euro-American psychiatry. (The implications of the term 'globalization' are discussed in Chapter 1; and the issues around the place of 'evidence-based medicine' (EBM) in the mental health field is discussed in Chapter 6.)

The funding sources of MGMH have not been disclosed. Money from the pharmaceutical industry may well be directly or indirectly involved because (a) Gates Foundation (which has funded many global *health* projects) states that it chose not to fund global *mental* health because NIMH-USA and the pharmaceutical industry already does so (Gates Foundation, 2010); and (b) a taught course for MSc. associated with MGMH organized by the London School of Hygiene and Tropical Medicine (LSHTM) in collaboration with King's College London Institute of Psychiatry (IOP) is supported to the tune of nearly £300,000 by Janssen Pharmaceutica (LSHTM, 2013), one of the major companies with vested interests in manufacture of psychotropic drugs.

In 2011, a special article in the prestigious international journal *Nature* (Collins *et al.*, 2011) described the processes that were being enacted to further the aims of MGMH. An initiative was launched to identify 'priorities for research' (p. 27)—the so-called 'Grand Challenges in Global Mental Health'. This project was backed by the US National Institute for Mental Health (NIMH-USA) and supported by the Global Alliance for Chronic Diseases (GACD), the former being a federal agency of the USA, and GACD a body hosted by University College London (UK) composed of organizations that aim to tackle the burden of chronic non-communicable diseases in LMICs (http://www.gacd.org/). Significantly, 'mental health' was defined as covering 'mental, neurological and substance use disorders' (p. 27). By mixing up categories (of illness) for which clear organic causes have been established with others that are largely convenient labels for a range of problems with social and/or psychological aetiology that may not be applicable universally (Chapter 2), such an approach muddies the waters all round of both research and service planning.

In order to pursue the Delphi method for identifying priorities for research (Jones and Hunter, 1995), an administrative team at NIMH-USA had solicited opinions from a number of 'experts' using unspecified procedures; and then a 'consensus' on priorities for research into global mental health was arrived at. The 'Delphi panel' of people nominated by NIMH-USA—as far as one can see—excluded obvious stakeholders among community workers, indigenous healers, religious organizations and service users in LMICs. Moreover, anecdotal reports indicated that the selection of the Delphi panel may well have been influenced by personal connections rather than objectively assessed 'expertise' of panel members (personal communication to author).

Opposition to MGMH

MGMH has been widely criticized. Campbell and Burgess (2012) of the London School of Economics comment:

> Whilst the Global Mental Health Movement's rhetoric and literature frequently refer to the need for greater community involvement, references to communities tend to be firmly located within the medical model of disease and recovery. Communities remain narrowly defined as patients and their families, and lay health workers linked to primary health care facilities. The lay health workers are viewed largely as handmaidens of biomedical expertise, with their role seen as that of helping in the scaling up of medically oriented mental health services. (p. 381)

An article in *Cultural Sociology of Mental Illness* states:

> Although the MGMH claims repeatedly to be 'evidence-based', critics point out that the 'evidence' it uses is selective and often dubious. Adequate research in LMI countries hardly exists, so that estimates of the global prevalence and burden of so-called 'MNS

disorders' have been based on arbitrary assumptions and unwarranted extrapolations.

(Ingleby, 2014, in press)

Two letters and two articles in Indian journals are seriously critical of the NIMH-USA approach in global mental health (Das and Rao, 2012; Shukla *et al.*, 2012a,b,c) one of which refers to the fact that a letter on the lines of the criticisms specified was rejected for publication by *Nature*. A neo-colonial analysis of the work of the MGMH shows how ideologies from the Global North are being imposed on the Global South (Mills, 2013); and the very idea that there is a globally valid concept called 'mental health' and that there are 'global' remedies for what amount to social suffering in LMICs has been criticized (Summerfield, 2012). Some of the speakers at a major meeting in Montreal in July 2012 highlighted the dangers posed to the Third World by MGMH (Bemme and D'souza, 2012).

What is most disturbing is not so much the apparent influence of NIMH-USA and GACD on MGMH but that MGMH may be supported by Big Pharma and that its approach appears to be getting support from North American funders calling for proposals for research to address grand challenges derived by the Delphi process. Individuals working in the MGMH and the people trained by it may well have good intentions but when powerful agencies dominate a movement, the outcomes are likely to be problematic—in a broad sense, 'neo-colonial'.

Promoting diagnoses

Whether it is a part of globalization (Chapter 1 for discussion of globalization) or not, the economic rise in the past decade of Brazil, Russia, India and China is resulting in changes impinging on health services in the developing world. As the middle class, who have the money and political influence in places like India and China, demand the 'best' from the West in the way of health care—invariably seen in terms of the latest technical advances—new imperatives arise in LMICs. Popular pressures determine government action and make demands on NGOs, which are now playing a major part in health development. And the pressures are often for developing the sort of services available in the West. As mental health is seen as being like any other type of 'health' in the arena of medicine—and that is the ideology that is being promoted by movements such as MGMH and even taken up by the media—the latest advances in remedies for mental health ill-health are assumed to be the latest drugs or the latest model of ECT machine. And the promotion of the use of diagnoses (whether they are based on ICD or DSM or in-between) opens the doors to the marketing of drugs by direct advertising or (more often) subtle means. In the course of recent visits to Sri Lanka, I came across the following situations that had occurred sometime around between 2007 and 2010.

Anecdote one: The camp approach to health education is well established and used to spread knowledge about infectious conditions such as tuberculosis and HIV. An INGO (international non-governmental organization), working in Sri Lanka at the time, adopted this approach as a part of developing educational programs on mental health by carrying out the following process: Initially, so-called 'community workers' were sent to a village armed with short symptom checklists which they used to identify people (allegedly) 'suffering' from one or other psychiatric illness. Then the people who had been identified as potential patients, together with their relatives, were invited to a 'camp' where they were given a lecture by a psychiatrist outlining the remedies available for the different diagnoses, and invited to partake of the drugs displayed on a table, or given by injection.

Anecdote two: An agency located abroad in a developed country, which had linked up with some local professionals after inviting them for paid-for 'training' in mental health work, proposed (through these local contacts) sending a team to 'train' community workers in Sri Lankan villages. The agency together with local contacts connected with the (governmental) mental health directorate to organize a public meeting to publicize their plan. It emerged at this meeting that the plan was to 'train' selected individuals in villages on how to diagnose 'depression', based on psychiatric models and symptom lists. A few weeks later, a local newspaper published its investigation into the foreign agency involved. Although it was officially a non-profit making organization, many of the people on its management were heavily involved in pharmaceutical companies and some of the professionals on its board specialized in lecturing on behalf of these companies to promote particular antidepressants. Once this was exposed by a local investigative journalist, the (governmental) mental health directorate pulled out of supporting this scheme which was to have been funded by the foreign agency.

The manoeuvres referred to above are examples of how psychiatric diagnosis and use of medication (closely linked together) are being promoted in the Third World. The end result of such manoeuvres is likely to be the opening of markets for neuroleptics marketed as anti-depressants, anxiolytics, anti-psychotics and so on. Another danger could well arise from the emergence of public–private partnerships (PPP) in the developing western-type mental health services in LMICs. A recent report (Nakimuli-Mpungu *et al.*, 2013) on the setting up of 'psycho-trauma centres' for 'delivering low-cost evidence-based mental health care' (p. 2) to people in Uganda via an arrangement between a public body and private organization (PPP scheme) praised the value of PPPs in raising funds. In this instance, it was not a pharmaceutical company that was involved but a foundation that trained people in western models of trauma-therapy; and the centres that were set up delivered 'psychopharmacology and psychotherapy' (p. 3) using DSM-IV criteria for diagnosis (APA, 1994).

Conclusions

The significant points that stand out in the international politics of mental health and psychiatry are summarized in Table 8.1. At a geopolitical level, policies in developing countries have been forced into abiding by neo-liberal ideologies allied to the powerful imperative of certain nations to be 'torch-bearers of an Anglo-American civilization' (Steger and Roy, 2010, p. 43). The result has been to increase disparities in wealth and health between the rich and poor countries of the world, and similar disparities within countries in both the Global South and the Global North. The focus on social determinants of health is a welcome development but WHO seems unable or unwilling to give a lead on tackling these. Meanwhile, NGOs and governments tend to/choose to ignore the need to address social determinants,

Table 8.1   Politics of mental health and psychiatry

Widespread adoption of neo-liberal policies
Interests of big business, especially pharmaceutical companies
Ignoring action on social determinants
Shifts in WHO policies—adopting western ideologies
Pressures to westernize (as 'globalization')
Myth of global remedies for mental health problems
Promoting psychiatric diagnoses in low- and middle-income countries

concentrating instead on providing (what they regard as) 'mental health services'—too often focused on 'treatments' available in HICs. WHO appears to have changed its tune during the past two decades; from being sensitive to the notion of mental health as a variable concept across cultures, covering a wide range of problems largely of a social and psychological nature, to backing the promotion of a bio-medical diagnosis-based approach to mental health development in LMICs. Thus WHO appears to support a movement that promotes westernization (as 'globalization') and the ideology that there are 'global' remedies for mental ill health available in 'evidence based' medicine of western psychiatry and that these should be spread across the world by popularizing traditional psychiatric diagnoses.

Many countries in the Global South have a wide range of needs not just for personal mental health and social care (equivalent roughly to personal and community well-being and access to help when in trouble and suffering distress) but also for stability of communities torn apart by recent wars and invasions, not to speak of recovery from the aftermath of prolonged colonialism. In such a context, medicalization of ordinary (understandable) anxieties and depressions re-constructed as personal illness can only result in exacerbating what Kirmayer (2006) has identified as 'the danger that focusing attention on mental health needs only serves to divert attention from more difficult social problems that demand political and economic solutions' (p. 138). And even more importantly, by promoting the use of drugs as remedies for personal problems conceptualized as 'illnesses', the medicalization process associated with marketing of neuroleptics is undermining indigenous, culturally acceptable means of help and support for people with personal or social problems resulting in distress. Subtle marketing of neuroleptics in LMICs is undoubtedly taking place often through promoting the use of psychiatric diagnoses to describe problems of living and personal distress—apart that is of pressures and inducement being brought to bear on professionals in LMICs who prescribe drugs and on governments to popularize psychiatry (see Khan, 2009). Big business may well look to profit in the future through PPP arrangements as much as by direct marketing of drugs.

A question that was raised and left hanging in the air at the end of the morning of a conference at Montreal in 2012 discussing 'global mental health' (referred to above) projected the feeling among several members of the audience (mainly from the Global North) that whatever the problems, the West, the rich nations, the Global North, should *do something* to promote better mental health services in the Global South. I think that in some ways the feeling is reciprocated in the South and also underlies the personal motivations of many of the people who work in organizations such as WHO and INGOs. But what is clear is that mental health development that consists of 'scaling up' services in LMICs to match those in HICs may do immense damage globally and should be resisted, especially since current systems in the West are far from being fit for purpose (Chapter 7). Chapter 9 suggests ways in which services in the West may be improved; and Chapter 10 suggests ways of local development that could improve the mental health and well-being of people living in LMICs and provide them with appropriate and sustainable mental health services.

Part IV

Developing Mental Health Services

Taking on board the complexities involved in what 'mental health' means today in a world where traditional cultures are becoming hybridized and political and economic forces impinge on mental health service provision, Part IV suggests changes in mental health services in the Global North that could be instituted without too much upheaval; and then proposes ways of developing mental health and well-being services in the Global South in an ethical and sustainable manner, suited to the needs of the people concerned. The ultimate requirement in both North and South is for services to be derived from *local* thinking, developed bottom-up and home-grown.

9

Modernizing Mental Health Services in the Global North

Chapter 8 discussed the state of play in mental health in the Global North and the way the Euro-American mental health system, with its bio-medical psychiatry, is being spread across the world. This chapter considers how mental health services in the West, mainly looking at UK and North America, could be updated and modernized to meet the needs of its multicultural society, conscious of the need to involve at all levels people who use services—'nothing about us without us' (Charlton, 2000). My personal experience has been primarily in the British National Health Service (NHS) that is funded by general taxation and free at the point of access to all who use it; and I have very limited knowledge of services in the private sector in the UK and even less of services in North America. In my travels and discussions with professionals outside the UK, I have surmised that the organization and delivery of mental health services in some parts of Europe and North America, such as The Netherlands and Canada, although resourced via insurance schemes, seem to be experienced in ways similar to those in UK—essentially available free to all who use them. Therefore, the suggestions for change made in this chapter, although specifically geared to suit NHS services and draw on my knowledge of these over many years, apply elsewhere in Euro-America too, although not in the private (for-profit) sector. The changes I suggest are relatively simple and practical, and do not necessarily challenge the basic structure of the mental health system or, to any great extent, the ways in which psychiatry functions. I have purposely not addressed any major re-ordering nor do I suggest a radical paradigm shift in psychiatry as envisaged, for example, in the special article in the *British Journal of Psychiatry* by Bracken *et al.* (2012), but stay with alterations and shifts that could eventually lead to major changes in service provision.

Starting with a short analysis of the basic faults in current practices that can be changed without too much upheaval the chapter goes on to consider ways of redressing inequality; changing legislation in the UK (limited to England, Wales and Northern Ireland because Scotland has somewhat different mental health legislation); collaboration between providers and users of services; improving the quality of multidisciplinary team-work and scope of treatments provided; regulating the pharmaceutical industry; and finally implementing a system where the concept 'well-being' replaces the primary place occupied by 'mental health' and where the recovery approach formulated by service users becomes central to service provision.

What can be changed?

In the past I have made several attempts to define broad-based changes that could improve mental health services in UK, especially with an eye on redressing inequalities arising from issues of racism and cultural insensitivity. My very first book (Fernando, 1988) about mental health services in UK was mainly about the practice of psychiatry and ended with the chapter 'A Blue-print for Change'. I wrote about 'de-politicisation' and freeing the discipline of psychiatry from its racist and oppressive history; and enabling mental health services to operate with equity in an unequal world. That was 25 years ago. Times are different. Clearly change is still required but (in my view) it is not merely change in psychiatric practice (in the narrow sense I saw it 25 years ago) that we should strive for. Psychiatry itself as an institution or discipline is in crisis (Chapter 6) but still occupies a fairly powerful position in the western world. As Will Self (2013) the British writer puts it in a popular newspaper: 'Just as we are quietly grateful to prison officers for banging up criminals, so too we are grateful for psychiatrists and psychiatric nurses for providing a cordon sanitaire between us and flamboyant insanity' (p. 2). Also (in the West) the illness-definitions that psychiatry provides still underpin much of the work done within health and social care services which are undoubtedly where many people turn to for help for a variety of problems. So changing these services for the better is what we should aim for—with an eye on the fact that how we do things here (in the Global North) is likely to influence, if not determine, one way or another the services that develop in the Global South (see Chapter 10).

Looking at mental health services in England (and assuming that they resemble services in other parts of the western world) the basic

Table 9.1   Basic faults in mental health services

Lack humanity—for example, ignore spirituality and values
Experienced as oppressive
Ignore the voice of service users
Too focused on diagnosis implying bio-medical dysfunction
Look too often to the 'magic pill'

faults that I detect from personal experience and by talking to people who have used mental health services are that, today, these services (Table 9.1) to a large extent:

(a) Lack humanity—often expressed as not being interested in spirituality, devoid of values and treating people as 'things'. Clearly many professionals in the services act humanely and with compassion, but the system does not encourage such ways of working.

(b) Tend to be oppressive—something seen in terms of high levels of compulsory detention especially of people seen as 'the other' nearly always identified in racial terms (see Chapter 7).

(c) Ignore the voice of service users who often have ideas derived from personal experience about how services should be organized and, even more importantly, on what they need from the services.

(d) Are too focused on encapsulating the problems presented by service users within diagnoses based merely on symptoms elicited by standard procedures, thereby missing issues in their life situations. However, I think that most people who use services are mostly concerned (when they access services) about getting effective help with what they perceive as their psychological problems than in worrying about the way assessments (of their needs) are made or the theories that professionals hold about health and illness.

(e) Look far too often to the 'magic pill' to cure illness thereby ignoring the realities of people's lives. This reflects the extent to which drug-based psychiatry (Chapter 6) has permeated mental health services as a whole.

Unfortunately I have not detected any important over-arching ideas from academic research that could inform the direction that changes in mental health services (already established in basic structure) should pursue. The role played by social determinants of health in causing social and personal suffering across the world is well recognized (Chapter 8) and the importance of social inequality in causing the

Table 9.2 Modernizing mental health in the Global North

Redressing inequalities
Changing legislation
Service-user involvement
Less hierarchical team-work
Joint inter-professional training
Widen scope of treatment
Controlling the pharmaceutical industry
Well-being recovery as a model for service provision

---

very high rates of depressions and anxieties in western countries has been highlighted recently (Wilkinson and Picket, 2010). Addressing these social determinants effectively involves political action, rather than changes in mental health services as such—at least in the way they are structured in advanced industrialized countries. (It may be different for the Global South—see Chapter 10.) For rich countries with firmly entrenched systems of mental health service provision, the main inequalities that could be addressed in mental health services (without necessarily interventions in wider society) are those around racism and cultural sensitivity (Chapter 7). The next few paragraphs discuss some of these matters summarized in Table 9.2.

Inequalities

There have been many attempts in the UK to redress some of the racial and cultural inequalities mentioned in Chapter 7. Some of these attempts have been covered elsewhere (Fernando, 1995, 2005; Fernando and Keating, 2009a). One of the earliest approaches at a clinical level was the 'cultural consultation' approach. In the late 1970s, Philip Rack, the local psychiatrist at Lynfield Mount Hospital at Bradford (Yorkshire) set up a multicultural team of professional staff, including religious leaders, that spanned 'a wide range of cultural as well as personal and professional backgrounds' (Rack, 1982, p. 268). The team provided consultative advice to their colleagues (providing mental health services) on cultural aspects of clinical care and also ran outpatient clinics for people of (mainly) Pakistani-Asian and Polish backgrounds living in the vicinity of the hospital. Similar arrangements were made in a few other places in the UK; for instance, I was involved with colleagues at Chase Farm Hospital in Enfield (Middlesex) during the mid-1980s onwards (until I left the services there in 1993) in providing cultural consultation on patients of the mental health unit at the hospital, but not taking over their care (as happened in Bradford). In the past decade, this approach, set up in a more elaborate fashion where consultation was backed by academic input by anthropologists, has been reported from Montreal (Canada) (Kirmayer *et al.*, 2003) and also from a teaching hospital in London (UK) (http://www.culturalconsultation.org.uk/). In fact, informal cultural consultation is provided by individual psychiatrists and psychologists interested in transcultural issues to their colleagues in many places in UK and some non-governmental agencies (in UK) too sometimes provide this type of service to the statutory sector on an informal basis.

Although cultural consultation services help professionals to remedy gross mistakes in cultural understanding (and hence no doubt help patients to feel accepted and understood by people providing the service concerned), in my view, they have a very limited impact on redressing inequality in service provision; consultation services, because of their focus on individual cases (the management of individual patients by the professionals involved), do not address issues of institutional discrimination, insensitivity and racism. In fact, institutional racism may be rendered more difficult to counteract sometimes when there is a cultural consultation service to hand, the presence of the latter tending to obscure what is happening below the surface of case management. Specialist services too are of limited value to the service provision as a whole because they have little effect on the general run of mental health services, although often valued by individual service users and their relatives who access them. The main attempts in the UK to address what is often called 'race inequality' in mental health services (Chapter 7) have been (a) top-down re-structuring through interventions at various levels of service provision, the last such plan being 'Delivering Race Equality' (DOH, 2005), and (b) educational approaches, such as 'race equality and cultural capability (RECC) training' (Ferns, 2009, p. 108) aimed at changing professional practices within the NHS. Unfortunately very little change has resulted from either approach for several reasons, the main ones (discussed by Fernando and Keating, 2009a) being around the power of (western) psychiatry and psychology in dominating the mental health system coupled with the fact that institutionalized racism requires wider interventions in society than mere alterations in the way mental health services are delivered.

In the UK, many initiatives for providing mental health care and advocacy in the community outside the statutory services have come and gone over the years, some highly appreciated by people who used them but few surviving more than three or four years because of problems over funding. Most have never been reported in the public domain; but some of those written up about five years ago (Fernando and Keating, 2009b) are still active although somewhat changed in scope: Family therapy in Asian and Chinese languages provided at the Marlborough Family Service in London (Malik *et al.*, 2009); counselling and day care for Asian, mainly Muslim, people at Qalb Centre in East London (Choudhry and Bakhsh, 2009); counselling and support for African-Caribbean people at a centre in Manchester (Stanley, 2009); and a variety of services for Chinese people in several parts of the UK (Au and Tang, 2009).

In the current political climate in the UK (and possibly most of Euro-America) specific action at a governmental level to counteract inequality in mental health services is unlikely, at least in the short term. Hence it seems best to look to shifts of emphasis in services (discussed below) through legislation, service user participation and so on.

Legislation

The laws in the UK vis-à-vis mental health and illness have been updated over the past 100 years moving in successive changes of legislation towards improving safeguards against excessive use of compulsory treatment and greater recognition of the rights of people designated as 'mentally ill'. That is until changes in the Mental Health Act for England and Wales that resulted in the current Mental Health Act (2007) (MHA), which went against history by widening the definition of mental disorder and so extending the range of people liable to compulsory treatment, while at the same time increasing the importance of risk assessments in decision-making by professionals (for fuller discussion of the negative effect of changes in legislation, see Inyama, 2009). In 2007 however, the Mental Capacity Act (2005) (MCA) came on the statute books providing for medical treatment to be given compulsorily if someone lacks capacity to make the decisions about need for medical treatment and stipulating a process for establishing 'capacity'. In this confused legal situation (of two laws that could apply in the field of mental health), 'mental health law based on risk... [is allowed] ... to "trump" mental health law based on capacity and individual autonomy' (Owen *et al.*, 2009, p. 258)—in other words if the MHA is applicable in any given situation, that must take precedence over the MCA. From human rights perspective, capacity-based legislation (as in MCA) is preferable to risk-based legislation (as in MHA) and much more likely to promote equity in mental health service provision. Therefore, services would be much improved—as well as more in tune with human rights—if the current MHA is repealed (abolished), so that the MCA is applied in the mental health field. Such a change will remove the centrality of risk-assessment in professional practice in mental health work and enable supportive relationships to play a greater part in service provision.

An alternative to complete abolition of the MHA—something that the general public may find difficult to support—is to revise selected parts of the MHA to ensure that the MCA can be used in preference to the MHA in specific circumstances when compulsory care or treatment is being considered. Or else, specific changes can be made in the MHA—an indication of how this could be done is contained in recommendations made by black and minority ethnic groups in the UK in the lead up to the legislative changes that were implemented in 2007. The recommendations, contained in official letters to the Department of Health, included the following (Inyama, 2009, pp. 37–8): (a) That legislation should make it legally binding for any detaining authority (instituting compulsory detention for treatment) 'to consult with such persons, appropriate community organizations and human rights bodies as have knowledge of patient's social and cultural background' (p. 37). (b) That, in the case of patients from black and minority ethnic communities, Approved Mental Health Professionals (AMHPs) (people who have authority over patients who are compulsorily detained in hospital or subject to community treatment orders) should have skills that are appropriate for working in a multicultural society (to be defined in legislation). (c) That the judgement of the presence or absence of mental disorder for purposes of compulsory detention and/or enforcement of treatment should take account of the patient's social and cultural background; and a legally binding statement to be included to ensure that mental disorder should not be construed by reason only of culturally appropriate beliefs and/or behaviour. (d) That any treatment given compulsorily should take account of the patient's culture, gender, sexuality and social background. And (e) that there is a legally binding provision for all service providers to abide by human rights and anti-discriminatory practice, the principles being modelled on those already within Scottish mental health legislation.

The suggestions listed above could fairly easily be added as amendments to current mental health legislation applicable to England and Wales. Although far short of what is required for addressing race inequality, action on these lines would establish the basis for further changes in the future as well as make a difference straight away.

Service user involvement

Although the importance of 'service user involvement', which is the involvement of people who use mental health services in a variety of ways in which the services operate, has been stressed in various official documents in the UK starting with the *National Service Framework for Mental Health* (DOH, 1999), but statements have been seldom matched by practice, at least not in ways that result in the service user voice having practical effect or even heard properly. Service users are often invited to planning meetings and consulted by managers of services but invariably their voice is rendered ineffective through service users being marginalized or disregarded in various ways (Linnett, 1999); it seems to be a matter of being seen but not heard. This could be rectified quite easily. Premila Trivedi (2009), an activist in the field and herself a user of mental health services, believes that there is an important role for service users 'in the development of mental health policy and practice, for example, in the planning, delivery and monitoring of mental health services, in the training and education of mental health staff and in mental health research' (p. 136).

The rights of service users to have influence in service planning should be either enshrined in law or at least given some teeth by a process whereby service user organizations can elect representatives on appropriate boards of management of services. In the 1980s, Mind (the National Association for Mental Health for England and Wales) recognizing the difficulty of incorporating the service user voice effectively at management level, decided to have two places on its Board of Management reserved for service users. In fact that manoeuvre was so successful that when Mind recognized a similar problem in the case of voices of ethnic minorities being heard, a similar system was established. It would be a fairly simple matter for Mental Health Trusts (in the case of UK's National Health Service), or similar boards of management of services for mental health, to ensure that suitable ways are devised for service users to be represented in management structures so that their voice has an impact on organization of services.

Team work, training and scope of treatment

Mental health services in the (British) NHS are supposed to be delivered by multidisciplinary teams. But there is usually a tacit assumption that in a hierarchy of influence (the pyramid) in a team, the psychiatrist or psychologist is at the top. Flattening of the authority pyramid is sometimes talked of but seldom implemented in practice. However, whatever form the pyramid takes, there seem to be variations in the way power works in mental health systems, not so much in terms of individuals over-riding others but the implied dominance arising from the level of remuneration (of individuals in a team) and even more importantly status of their training. Doctors generally carry more power through both these avenues when compared to other non-medical professionals in a multidisciplinary team. In my view, most people who are patients or clients would prefer to see the most important voice in a multidisciplinary team as that of the person (in the team) who knows them best, rather than the person who is paid the most or has had the longest training. How this is brought about in any one team is something for the team to decide but such change would certainly improve services.

In most NHS settings, treatment tends to focus on physical (as opposed to psychological) medical-type therapies, namly medication and sometimes ECT (electroconvulsive therapy) being the main ones. Other ways of helping people, such as counselling, psychotherapy and social support are seen as marginal to the main therapeutic programme. However, it was not always like that. For example, in the UK, both the crisis intervention movement, pioneered at Napsbury Hospital at St Albans (Scott, 1960), and the therapeutic community movement, most famously at Dingleton Hospital in Scotland (Jones, 1968) and Claybury Hospital in north-east London (Shoenberg, 1972), which were prominent in the late 1960s and 1970s (see Chapter 6), emphasized interpersonal relationships, social networks and family support as the basis of therapy. Even today, systemic approaches of family therapy (see Minuchin and Fishman, 1981) and some psychological therapies (see Haley, 1963) tend not to be based on a purely 'illness' approach to mental health problems, although most therapists using these approaches still adhere to the basic diagnostic medical model of psychiatry in selecting or accepting people for therapy. The perpetuation of narrow models for understanding and treating illness in most mainstream mental health services come partly from the fact that professional training is often in silos, each professional group being trained separately. Introducing joint training schemes could go some way in shifting current practice within teams toward a more flexible approach.

Widening the scope of treatments offered in mainstream mental health services, combined with service users being given a choice, is a way of moving forward into an age where psychiatry is multicultural. If service users are enabled to choose between several different types of therapy—and a variety of treatments are available—the present dissatisfaction with mental health services should be alleviated and inequality addressed to some extent. For this to happen, therapies from non-western cultural traditions need to be available, possibly by involving experts from non-western countries or their diasporas in the West. This would have the additional benefit of promoting interchange of knowledge and expertise between the Global South and the Global North (as suggested in Chapter 10).

Pharmaceutical industry

In her far-reaching and influential book *The Truth About the Drug Companies*, Marcia Angell (2005) former editor of the prestigious *The New England Journal of Medicine*, reviewed the excesses of drug company power exerted over many different health domains, including mental health. Today, the industry is often referred to as 'Big Pharma' (Law, 2006, title page) because of the power it seems to wield in the field of health, including mental health, not just by influencing prescribing habits of doctors, but also influencing political systems, medical education, and so on (Angell, 2005). One way that drug usage in the mental health field appears to have got out of control is well summarized in the quote: 'Once upon a time, drug companies promoted drugs to treat diseases. Now it is often the opposite. They promote diseases to fit their drugs' (Angell, 2005, p. 86). Chapter 6 discusses the 'medication revolution' in Euro-American psychiatry; the rise in numbers of disease categories listed in DSM and the rise of profits made by Big Pharma, as related events, have resulted in many of the current discontents with mental health services. And critiques of modern Euro-American psychiatry highlight the dependence in mainstream mental health services on what Moncrieff (2009) calls the 'myth of the chemical cure' (2009, title page). In trying to limit the use of medication in mental health services, it is essential to bring in some controls on the pharmaceutical industry. This can only be done through political means probably at a governmental level but limiting the use of drugs at the service provision level is also possible.

An approach to reducing the dependency of services on prescribing drugs would be educational. Increasing the information provided to professionals about a variety of alternatives to drugs, whether for controlling disturbed behaviour or for symptom relief, is one approach that may work, especially if followed up by feed-back on changes in practice as a result. Another would be the introduction of some regulation whereby a drug free period (say of one week) is made mandatory when anyone is taken on for treatment; or that a full report is called for if someone is prescribed drugs in preference to other treatments or at least when drugs are prescribed at a dosage higher than a specified level. In fact, I saw this manoeuvre used successfully in an acute ward of a mental hospital when I was a member of the Mental Health Act Commission and we (commissioners) had criticized some of the psychiatrists working in the ward for using excessive dosages of psychotropic medication. Finally, statutory obligation on prescribers of medication to provide up-to-date information on the dangers of whatever is prescribed could help. Clearly the particular approach at the level of interaction between prescribers and clients must be worked out by the multidisciplinary team concerned, but there is a role for management to ensure that service users and their relatives have all the information they need in order to question prescribers and to provide guidance and set targets.

Recovery and well-being

This section discusses two recent discourses that have become prominent in the mental health field in the West, namely 'recovery' that came to North America and UK from New Zealand, and 'well-being' from the field of mental health promotion (HEA, 1997) and community psychology (Diener, 1984; Nelson and Prilleltensky, 2005). Both have come about partly because of dissatisfaction with medical dominance of the mental health discourse felt by service users for a long time and more recently by many professionals in (western) psychology and even some psychiatrists (see, for example, discussions in Chapters 2 and 6); and also as a result of search by many people for some language through which they could make sense of emotional setbacks and ways of dealing with these in a meaningful way.

Recovery and the recovery approach

A prominent theme recently in mental health discourse in the UK and North America is 'recovery', the name given by the survivor/service-user movement to an alternative to the treatment and rehabilitation model (for illness) generally used in mental health services, and seen as a sort of journey to regaining a sense of purpose and self-worth after a major life disruption (Kloos, 2005). The journey following extreme distress or suffering (interpreted in psychiatry as illness) is not dependent on whether or not the people undertaking it receive 'treatment' as such; and the journey itself subsumes the pursuit of personal goals of maintaining hope, making sense of experiences, understanding and empowerment (Repper and Perkins, 2003). Allied to the concept of recovery is the term 'recovery approach' which is about the role of services and systems in supporting the journey of recovery. Unfortunately, this new imaginative approach has come up against a meaning of recovery that is well established in the medical literature, although it had got somewhat lost in psychiatry. Recovery in medical discourse is part of the western medical model of illness; the aim of medical (including psychiatric) treatment being either 'cure' and/or the promotion of recovery. So currently there are two definitions of recovery in the public discourse on mental health: First, the psychiatric one of the long-term goal of remission and/or control of symptoms; and second, the pursuit of personal goals (as described above) irrespective of the illness label. It is the latter (service-user constructed) model of recovery that I wish to pursue in this section.

In tracing the roots of the recovery movement in the mental health field, Davidson *et al.* (2010) find it in the late eighteenth century France when Philippe Pinel, together with Jean-Baptiste Pussin, an ex-patient and the manager of the asylum at Bicêtre, treated the inmates humanely with compassion and understanding, seeing 'mad' people as very special people who needed protection from society while they got over their affliction in their own time (Chapter 3). Davidson *et al.* (2010) see aspects of recovery also in (a) the immediate postcolonial period when people who had been subjugated and disempowered for many years began to take control over their own destinies by nation building; and (b) in the period after the 1960s civil rights struggles in USA, when African-Americans took control over their own lives, often fighting off institutionalized hostility. In the case of colonialism, once the colonizers decided to leave, the responsible thing that they should have done was to have provided a context for the new nations to recover, make their own choices, and take power into their own hands—a process analogous to the recovery journey of service users. In fact there was a half-hearted attempt to do something like that in British and French colonies in the approach to independence (Jones, 1983): The community development (CD) approach of participatory action research, and its counterpart *animation rurale*, designed to enable communities long disempowered to participate in development in various fields (including health care), were first used by Britain and France during the 1950s in some of their colonies heading towards independence (Macdonald, 1992). On the whole, these approaches failed to deliver because there was no real sharing of power between urban-centred governmental organizations that took over from colonial structures and the largely rural communities (Holdcroft, 1978).

The CD approach is a model for what mental health services *should* do in a recovery approach to support people on the journey of recovery. It is about partnership between service providers and service users to develop support networks, promote hope and enable integration of service users into the mainstream of wider society (social inclusion). Clearly, such support of the recovery journey (by service providers) has to be honest and responsible, not just an excuse for withdrawing support and help from people in need. Continuing to control and dominate ex-colonial countries (neo-colonialism) is wrong, just as colonization of minds seen as 'disordered' (by psychiatric interventions) and then not helping when the people who actually own the minds (the service users concerned) take control is wrong. There is a lesson there for mental health services on how people considered as 'patients' should be allowed to take over their own lives by working with professionals as partners.

Returning to the practicality of recovery in a multi-ethnic western society where psychiatry dominates the mental health scene, a problem in the recovery discourse so far is that it focuses too much on being an individualized process and that the meaning given to distress is one of illness—something that does not connect fully with service users from non-western cultural backgrounds (Kalathil, 2007). If it is to have meaning in a multicultural society, a recovery approach (a service approach that promotes recovery) must address the needs of people who feel oppressed in society at large as well as within the services; and the recovery journey being as much *social* as *personal*. It may be the case that, in such a context, recovery is too mild a word to encompass this journey towards a respectable and fulfilling life; liberation may be preferable. Also the pursuance of the recovery approach in service provision needs to grasp the reality that it is the service-user model and not the medical one that mental health services must address.

In summary, I suggest that recovery is about freedom, the eternal yearning for freedom that is probably inherent in human beings worldwide. For people who are undertaking the recovery journey, it is no longer about *surviving* the system (be it the psychiatric system or some other situation felt as oppressive) or just about surviving setbacks, crises or misfortunes that are the lot of all human beings; but it is about *recovering* from any or all of these. So services should no longer mainly be about treating or intervening in people's lives, following up to make sure people keep to their treatment, providing advice on what they can and should not do, and generally managing and directing 'patients' from a position of expertise backed by power. Services providing a recovery approach must be structured to enable the recovery journey to take place, supporting and providing a context that enables people to make their own personal choices and allow them to take power aver their lives into their own hands. In a real sense the recovery approach is about liberating people; allowing them to be free.

Well-being

The past decade has seen efforts to access the meaning attributed to mental health without referring to the word 'health', mainly to avoid dependency on 'experts' imposing their judgments and to enable people who use services to think for themselves. Also there has been a search for a word that avoids locating experience just 'in the head' (that the word 'mental' does) since most people identify their feelings as affecting their total self, getting away to some extent from the western tradition of Cartesian duality (Chapter 2). The search has been for language that reflects experience and feelings of people in a way that reflects meaningfully what they want from helping agencies and what they expect when they access a service meant to help them. Moreover, well-being seems to have emerged as a word that can be adequately translated into various languages (see below).

The use of well-being is justified in western psychology literature on the grounds that, in contrast to 'mental health', well-being (a) is based on standards and values chosen by people themselves; (b) reflects success or failure in achieving norms and values that people themselves seek; and (c) includes components 'dependent on pleasure and the fulfillment of basic human needs, but also includes people's ethical and evaluative judgments of their lives' (Diener and Suh, 2000, p. 4). At a personal level, well-being—sometimes called 'subjective well-being' (SWB) (Diener, 1984; Diener and Suh, 2000)—is a positive state of affairs brought about by satisfaction of personal, relational and collective needs (Prilleltensky et al., 2001). When community perceptions of well-being are accessed in community psychology and development studies, these individual components are added to by 'the synergy created by all of them [personal, relational and collective needs] together' (Nelson and Prilleltensky, 2005, p. 56).

Well-being (as defined by people themselves), translated into local languages, has been used for many years in qualitative action research, especially in the group of processes subsumed under 'Participatory Rural Appraisal' (PRA) and 'Rapid Rural Appraisal' discussed in the book *Whose*

Reality Counts? Putting the First Last (Chambers, 1997). On well-being Chambers (1997) writes:

> *The objective of development is well-being for all.* Well-being can be described as the experience of good quality of life. Well-being and its opposite ill-being differ from wealth and poverty. Well-being and ill-being are words with equivalents in many languages. Unlike wealth, well-being is open to the whole range of human experience, social, mental and spiritual as well as material.
>
> (1997, pp. 9–10, italics in original)

A recent project in Sri Lanka found that the term 'well-being' in its Tamil and Sinhala language equivalents enabled the researchers to explore feelings and experiences in a meaningful, sensitive and effective fashion (discussed in Chapter 10).

Discussions around the concepts of recovery and well-being have been going on for some considerable time in UK and North America. The confusion resulting from the subtle power struggle over the use of the term 'recovery'—between professional psychiatric systemic power of the medical establishment and the voice of service users and like-minded people—needs to be called off, enabling the service user viewpoints to stand. Then the two concepts, well-being and recovery, could form an alternative to the diagnosis-treatment approach of traditional bio-medical psychiatry—to the betterment of psychiatric practice and mental health service provision generally (see Fernando *et al.*, 2013).

Conclusions

Radical change in the structure of mental health services in the Global North and/or a paradigm shift in psychiatry may occur one day in the future, but in the short term relatively minor changes could make a difference to service users and get the ball rolling for major changes to come. I have outlined the changes that may work in the British NHS hoping these may be applicable in essence all over the Global North to a greater or lesser extent. In looking to the more distant future, some of the answers—at least at the 'soft end' of psychiatry that associates with the disciplines of clinical psychology, counselling and psychotherapy in providing various 'talking therapies' (forms of psychological therapy)—may come from innovations that are currently being tried out in various places in the UK (and I expect in other parts of the world). One particular approach is to develop multicultural therapy by combining in practical ways religious approaches to counselling with more traditional (western) therapy. These and other mixtures may eventually surface in what in some parts of UK are vibrant inclusive multicultural communities. Unfortunately, the future at the 'hard end' of psychiatry where people are compulsorily detained and often harshly treated (which is where many people from racial minorities end up), the future does not look very promising. The resolution of the problems there appears to lie in political change outside mental health itself.

10

Mental Health and Well-Being in the Global South

The topic of mental health development in low- and middle-income countries (LMICs) is complicated: They are largely non-western in cultural background (see Chapter 1 for discussion of culture); many were colonized by western powers in the past (see Chapter 5 for discussion of colonial psychiatry†) and some still struggle with postcolonial problems resulting in civil conflict, not to speak of neo-colonial economic domination (see Chapter 8); and, on the whole, they have a multiplicity of fields where development is required. In reality it is artificial and probably not all that productive to separate 'mental health' development from development in general. It is important to keep in mind too that the language of 'mental health' and 'mental illness' that we use in discussing development is embedded in western culture, the concepts themselves being derived from the study of madness as understood in the West, and so the discourse on 'mental health' is beset by problems of cultural translation and mistranslation (Chapter 2). Finally, unlike 'development' during colonial times (when the benefit was mainly for the colonial power concerned), development in a postcolonial world must be primarily for the benefit of local people in LMICs and geared to *their* cultural and social expectations. Yet, I concede that compromises may be required in the real world, mainly because some of the resources (in the form of investment) and some of the know-how for development has to come from high-income countries (HICs) and also because there is undoubtedly much that LMICs can learn from the way things are done in the developed world in many fields of health; for example, in general medical services such as HIV and tuberculosis. However, it must be borne in mind that *mental* health (*health* of the *mind*) is not just a *medical* matter (something repeatedly argued in this book, especially in various part of Chapters 2, 3, 6 and 7); in the case of LMICs in particular, social and cultural dimension (of mental health) may well be much more important than the medical.

In thinking of ways of developing mental health services in LMICs, the basic approach should be to (a) build on what there is now, changing the structures where necessary (for example, running down the asylums and regulating activities in other systems such as religious healing); (b) learning from experiences in the past and from what happens in other places all over the world; and (c) ensuring that the services that result are what the people of the countries concerned wish to have and that they are sustainable.

Three points should be noted to start with: First, culture, whether of individuals or communities, is never static but in a state of dynamic change. Although there has been hybridization of cultures, fundamental differences exist worldwide in terms of worldviews, ideologies about health and illness and the way matters to do with 'mind' are conceptualized (Chapter 1). Second, very different cultural traditions around mental health have emerged across the world, but these have not always remained very distinct from each other and certainly the differences between them have not necessarily remained unchanged over the years (Chapter 2). Third, although concepts and ideologies about mental health and illness have spread as a result of pressures and power imbalances (not to speak of direct imposition during colonial domination) mainly from the Global North to the Global South (Chapters 4, 5, 6 and 7), there is a need in development to redress the inequities that have resulted from such a one-sided movement, for example, the underdevelopment of indigenous medical and healing systems of the South. In other words, there is a need during development to ensure a level playing field for North–South interaction and this may involve protecting the Global South from potentially damaging systems being pushed on it by business interests and other forces that may be called (broadly speaking) neo-colonialism. Of course (but to a much lesser extent), ideas and knowledge about mental health have spread the other way too, from South to North. This South–North movement needs to be promoted and given prominence because it has been undervalued in the past. Fourth, mental health being intricately involved with ways of life, social conditions and life experiences of people concerned, it is important in development to address what is known about social determinants of health generally (Chapter 8).

A problem for planners in LMICs is that there is a lack of reliable information on effective and culturally appropriate systems for mental health care in LMICs. In the absence of hard data on what services and types of service structure are best suited to (culturally) non-western countries, the temptation is to look for an evidence base in research articles published in psychiatric literature. But this could be very misleading since these articles and reports (mainly in more recent times referring to randomized control trials of drug therapies) (a) invariably use (western) diagnostic systems which are not applicable in non-western settings; (b) ignore the limitations of the existing corpus of studies (Gupta, 2007) which, for example, disregard 'individual and collective experience as sources of knowledge' (Kirmayer, 2012, p. 253) thereby downgrading the knowledge inherent in the diverse cultural inheritances of people across the world, but mainly the non-western world; and (c) are often biased towards highlighting needs of people in HICs and organizational structures that suit western societies.

To repeat bits from Chapters 4 and 7: (a) The large study carried out in the 1970s called International Pilot Study of Schizophrenia (IPSS) (Chapter 7) seemed to indicate that the context for recovery from severe mental illness may have been better in *non-western* settings compared to western ones in the 1960s and 1970s, at a time when the influence of psychiatry in the Global South was weak; and (b) studies in India suggest that religious healing centres may be beneficial for people with serious mental illness (to use psychiatric jargon) and that providing a plurality of systems which service users and relatives could choose from may be conducive to high recovery rates of people with 'serious mental illness' (Chapter 4).

Considering the problems there are in carrying out valid international research (Chapter 4), it is very unlikely that psychiatry-based research (such as epidemiological studies using psychiatric diagnosis) would yield useful information for mental health development in the Global South; and resources should not be wasted in pursuing such research. Also, anthropological studies using ethnographic methods (as they are often carried out currently) are of limited value for service development because their findings are difficult to apply in developing mental health services except to provide some understanding of how people concerned perceive 'mental health' (and what might constitute mental ill-health) and what function they see for services. However, there is a need for research into matters neglected in the past; the sort of research required is exemplified by pilot studies carried out in Sri Lanka on current perceptions of mental illness in villages (Perera and Hettiarachchi, 2011) idioms of distress (Sivayokan, 2011) and treatment for mental illness provided by indigenous medical practitioners (Perera, 2011).

The diversity of the global scene in mental health and psychiatry as it exists today is not easy to address for the purpose of mental health development without discussing the use of the prefix *western*. Clearly, *western* psychiatry operates as part of western (or allopathic) medicine that arose in Europe and then spread to European settlements in North America, Australia and other parts of the world and, to varying extent, to (culturally) non-western regions of the world. These are rightly seen as a part of *western* culture. However, whether we like it or not, whether we regret what has happened or not, the fact-on-the ground is that 'westernization' sometimes masquerading as 'globalization' (see Chapter 1 for discussion of these terms) has taken place over the past 50 years, especially in the past two decades, whereby psychiatric thinking has penetrated the Global South to some extent, although often to limited sections of the people (Chapter 7). Today, we see western-type mental health services being installed in the Global South, although still mainly in urban areas; and psychiatry and western psychology being taught in universities all over the world. Yet there is no evidence that fundamental ideologies appertaining to mental health that are held by most people in LMICs, and the sort of philosophies most ordinary people in the non-western LMICs live by, have become westernized to any great extent. As with Coca-Cola and McDonald's, people may partake of what is available but still demur at a fundamental level preferring their own traditional ways of thinking about the human condition and hence their beliefs about health, illness and ideas about 'mind' (see discussions in Chapters 2, 4, 5 and 7).

While it is true that there appears often to be a common language around mental health among professionals and academics, especially evident in discourses in learned journals and international meetings across the world, I doubt that this common language applies to the vast majority of people. What appears to have happened is that sociocultural and economic barriers appear to have arisen between the professional and social elites in the Global South on the one hand, and the majority of the population of LMICs on the other, corresponding approximately to the class divides within each region as described by Navarro (2007). As a result, there is a commonality of interests, and a sort of limited common culture, between dominant classes in both the Global North and Global South (see Chapter 7). But fundamental cultural divisions between different peoples vis-à-vis matters to do with 'mind', mental health, and, in many ways, the nature of the human condition still exists, and likely to do so indefinitely. In other words, cultural diversity worldwide is a reality, a unicultural world is a state that can never be, possibly because of the nature of humankind as sociocultural beings.

It is evident from arguments in Chapter 8 that the discourse in all health considerations should focus on social determinants of health as well as on individual distress and ill-health. In other words, there should be two main components of mental health development, one largely political that acts on the knowledge there is about social determinants of health and one largely operational (practical, on the ground) in terms of relieving mental distress of individuals. This chapter argues that in general the former should be developed *top-down* and the latter *bottom-up*. However the two streams clearly overlap and meet at various points. For example, if one of the social determinants, say poverty, is tackled in a particular region or country, the services on the ground that would be needed there are likely to change, not only because poverty itself may cause mental distress but it also because poverty impedes people's ability to seek out mental health services they may benefit from.

This chapter discusses first, the current ground realities that we need to consider when discussing mental health development in LMICs. Next, I try to establish what the ground rules should be in development, leading naturally on to discuss how North–South collaboration can be promoted. A short section on community development appropriate to ground realities leads to discussing how the knowledge of social determinants of health should be mobilized to formulate national policies that could be followed through with practical action. Finally the concluding section of this chapter brings together the matters explored earlier to describe how best to go about developing mental health services in a two-pronged approach, top-down and bottom-up, in close consultation with communities concerned and basically home-grown.

It is true that many countries in the Global South do not have effective legislation defining responsibilities of service providers and rights of people receiving services in the field of mental health. This situation surely leads to injustices and must be remedied. However, in many of these countries there is a problem around implementation of laws and regulations. Introducing legislation of the type available in HICs of the West, such as the Mental Health Act (2007) in the UK, in the absence of properly organized services and an infrastructure to support implementation of the laws would only result in confusion and frustration for both providers and users of services. The priority is to get some of the services in place—legislation can come afterwards or as services are being brought into play so that laws and regulations are in line with what is available and that they (the laws) are feasible in practice. For this reason,

I have decided not to discuss the question of mental health legislation in LMICs but consider briefly what sort of regulation in particular situations may be required to help service development to proceed. Another matter not addressed (except briefly referred to under North–South collaboration and in the concluding section) is the issue of resources for development. The practical importance of this is undoubted but must be left for other works to explore.

Ground realities

In the context of cultural differences between the Global North and South, some people (for example, Summerfield, 2012) maintain that even the idea of *mental* health is a Eurocentric one that does not fit well into meeting needs of most people in non-western settings where the approach to health in general is holistic (rather than reductionist) (see Chapter 2). In my view, this is indeed so but, for better or worse, there has been some cultural shift in LMICs over the past three or four decades; the 'mental' idea has caught on to some extent and a limited reductionist 'illness' approach is not unknown—just as there seems to be some suggestions that the holistic idea is catching on in Europe and North America although to a much lesser extent (and I suggest in Chapter 9 that it should be promoted). In other words, cultural hybridity renders the term 'mental health' understandable worldwide (or almost worldwide) although it has different emphases and often given different meanings in different places. Also, development is a practical proposition, and for any practical process to be successful, compromises are necessary in the language used.

Mental health development in the Global South should not be seen as something separate from development in general, especially development that is aimed at poverty reduction and empowerment of people at the bottom of the pile socially and politically. In a series of studies across the Third World tapping into views and experiences of over 200,000 poor men, women, youth and children in 23 LMICs, the book *Voices of the Poor; Crying out for Change* (Narayan *et al.* 2000) states:

> Wellbeing and illbeing are states of minds and being. Wellbeing has a psychological and spiritual dimension as a mental state of harmony, happiness and peace of mind. Illbeing includes mental distress, breakdown, depression and madness, often described by participants to be impacts of poverty. (p. 21)

Thus, the concept of well-being is far better than 'mental health' for integrating mental health development with development in general geared to poverty reduction. Between 2007 and 2011, I was involved in a research programme in Sri Lanka (Weerackody and Fernando, 2008, 2011) conducted using 'a family of approaches and methods' that were community based and subsumed under 'participatory rural appraisal' (PRA) (Chambers, 1997, p. 102). 'Well-being' is one of the central constructs in PRA research that takes as its starting point the personal realities of individuals. The concept 'well-being' used in its Tamil and Sinhala language equivalents proved (in our studies consulting people from all main ethnic groups in the country) to be closely connected with the concept 'mental health' which I know so well in western psychology and psychiatry—and which was familiar to several of the bilingual/trilingual researchers in the Sri Lankan studies. The idea (concept) of 'well-being' was used to access a holistic approach to mental health seen as 'denoting material advancement, social aspirations, sense of security, and health seen as physical, mental and moral dimensions... [covering both]... subjective feelings and external circumstances', all experienced as a 'whole'—'holistically'—and not as separate 'factors' (Weerackody and Fernando, 2008, p. 55). Approaching well-being from a social science, developmental perspective connected well with well-being seen from a (western) psychological perspective. For these reasons, I suggest that in talking of developing mental health services in the Global South it is better to think more broadly of services for mental health *and* well-being as a combination. In fact, this connects with one of my suggestions for changes required in the Global North (Chapter 9). However there are several other ground realities considered in the next few paragraphs (Table 10.1).

Although health services in the West are geared mainly to alleviating mental distress seen as problems of personal illness largely located in the minds of individual human beings, and mind seen as brain activity, there is no evidence that this ideology is present to any great extent in the Global South. The basic emphasis on community over the individual, evident in pre-colonial Asia and Africa is still the dominant mode in most LMICs (see Chapters 2 and 4 and see Triandis, 1995 for discussion of individualism and collectivism). For example, in Northern Sri Lanka the effect on (mental) health of people caught up in armed conflict and affected by natural disasters was that they experienced 'collective trauma' (Somasundaram, 2007) rather than the individualized 'trauma' represented in the illness described in psychiatry Post Traumatic Stress

Table 10.1   Ground realities in planning services

Services should be for mental health *and* well-being
Need for a communitarian emphasis
    Community-based services
Limitations of western models and systems
    Ideologies of health and illness very different
    Evidence base from the West does not apply
    Learn from mistakes elsewhere
Look to local traditions, note local conditions and draw on diversity of
    knowledge
    Prioritize indigenous systems
    Draw on knowledge of systems elsewhere
    Plurality of services
Lack of social welfare, lack of regulation of services and sale of drugs
Poor public health infrastructure, inappropriate training of professionals
Context of geopolitical forces and neo-liberal policies
    Need for regulation of multinational corporations

Disorder (PTSD). Collective trauma denotes experiences such as disruption of trust among people and changes in significant relationships, rather than the 'symptoms' described (in psychiatry) as individualized mental disturbance. A point of relevance here is that, unlike the 'illness' PTSD (which is understood in terms of symptoms), the nature of 'collective trauma' can only be understood in terms that are specific to the particular society concerned; it can only be extracted and addressed bottom-up (by asking communities and groups to explore how the traumatic events affected them) and will be missed by a mental health service geared to models of individualized illness. There is little doubt that community-based (rather than institution-based) services would be more consistent with communal cultures of LMICs; and if these are developed to add on to the asylums already there from colonial times (hopefully regulated and cut down on size), a mixture of institutional and community-based services would eventually result— as in the West where this mixed model is now preferred (Thornicroft and Tansella, 2004).

As discussions in Chapters 2 and 3 on how claims of scientific respectability came about, and in Chapter 6 on the limitations of 'evidence-based medicine' (EBM) and alleged scientific basis for bio-medical psychiatry show, it is foolish to look *primarily* to western models of service provision for guidance on developing mental health systems in non-western settings, although some aspects of western models may well have relevance. It is important first and foremost to draw from cultural histories and traditions in LMICs themselves, keeping in mind the cultural diversity of what 'mental health' means (Chapters 2 and 4) and, above all, to listen to local voices so that services are geared to what people in these countries want and value. Careful study of what has happened in Euro-American model of psychiatry may provide knowledge of what precautions need to be taken to avoid the mistakes in the West. The unfortunate attitude sometimes prevalent among those in power in LMICs of turning to the West whenever development is considered may reflect a legacy of colonialism—what Homi Bhabha (1994), quoting the work of Frantz Fanon, calls the 'colonial condition' (p. 41) described in Chapter 5 and referred to in Chapter 7. Hence it is important to prioritize very consciously indigenous systems of care and help in planning services.

The fact that many ordinary people access—and seem to benefit from—a variety of therapies for (what psychiatrists may call) 'mental illness' (Chapter 4) is highly significant. It is important to note that poverty often limits ability of people to access services for there is little or no welfare support available from the state in most LMICs and whatever free services are supplied by the state are usually just drugs and/or ECT (electroconvulsive treatment). Indeed social welfare systems for supporting families in need may be one of the most effective ways of promoting access to services that people choose. Another ground reality to be faced in development is that there is very little regulation in most LMICs of whatever services are used by people concerned (whether religious, medical and so on) and of the sale of drugs; consequently, unethical and even dangerous practices (such as abuse of users of services or lack of fire-protection) may develop, and anyone can buy a drug (if available) so long as they know its name—or worse, they may sometimes be able to do so by providing a diagnosis. Of course the lack of regulation applies to all drugs and goes along with lack of controls on pharmaceutical promotion in LMICs (Lexchin, 1992); but in the case of neuroleptics, there are serious issues around their effectiveness, specificity and dangers (Chapter 6) as well as questions about the cross-cultural validity of psychiatric diagnosis allegedly treated by these drugs (Chapters 2 and 4). Unregulated availability of neuroleptics therefore carries particular drawbacks and the possible danger of promoting a drug-based culture in the society concerned—something that may profit Big Pharma but seriously damage the social fabric of the society concerned. Another reality that needs to be taken into account has been pinpointed by a psychiatrist in South India (Jacob, 2011) who is in close touch with community groups in his area; he points to the importance of addressing poverty, public health infrastructure, inappropriate training of mental health professionals including psychiatrists and the brain drain of professionals migrating to the West.

There are many individuals and groups in the Global North desirous of helping the South without imposing inappropriate (usually) western systems of mental health care and psychiatry but we need to be aware of political forces that have very different institutionalized 'intentions' (so to speak) loosely encapsulated in the term 'imperialism'. What actually happens in development may well be manipulated by business interests and geopolitical forces of various sorts. This may be a difficult problem to deal with in mental health development in the Global South and was discussed to some extent in Chapter 8. For, example, much of the financial resources necessary for development still comes from the West; and western agencies and funding bodies (that, for example, support NGOs working in the Global South), though officially independent and not influenced directly by big business, may nevertheless fulfil an imperial role; they may well be supported by donations from *for-profit* companies including pharmaceutical companies or they may unwittingly (or half-wittingly) promote ways of working that depend on medicalizing problems of living as issues of 'illness', thereby opening the doors in the Global South for Big Pharma to exploit; or they may support the advent of private health companies marketing their particular brand of 'evidence-based' treatment (see Chapter 6 for anecdotes that illustrate the subtle way in which drugs may be marketed and also for transcultural critiques of 'evidence based medicine', EBM).

Ground rules

Development is a seductive word that suggests a necessary path of progress. In colonial times, development was largely directed at producing cash crops and raw materials for manufacturing consumer goods in the West and providing markets for these in the colonies. Providing services for natives was often a mere by-product of the overall colonial project of extracting wealth and enabling political stability. In the immediate postcolonial period, development implied both social improvement and economic 'catching up' (Gasper, 2004, p. 35). But the discourse has moved on considerably since then. Much is made now of development in LMICs needing to be ethical and sustainable (Gasper, 2004; Warburton, 1998). We know that the imposition in colonial times of western-type asylums was a mistake; it did not really do much good and possibly helped towards underdevelopment of indigenous systems of mental health care (Chapter 5). Developing mental health systems in LMICs is not a simple matter of transferring established strategies used in HICs, irrespective of ground realities and ignoring the views of local people. Mental health is not just a technical matter but is tied up with ways of life, values, and worldviews that vary significantly across cultures and societies. In such a situation, ' "global thinking" is at best only an illusion and at worst the ground for... destructive and dangerous [local] actions' (Esteva and Prakash, 1997, p. 279). The approach that is required for mental health development in LMICs is *local* thinking, for a variety of reasons not least for cost-effectiveness, using the least resources to achieve the greatest gain (Kumaranayake and Walker, 2002). The first thing that planners should obtain is basic knowledge about local people. Then there are other rules that are equally important (Table 10.2).

Local knowledge

When services are being planned, planners should take on board as much local knowledge as they can obtain, such as information on local idioms of distress. Cultural variation in the way personal subjective distress is expressed is well established (Kirmayer, 1989; Kohrt and Hruschka, 2010; Nichter, 1981, 2010; Pedersen *et al.*, 2010). In addition, these may well be altered as a result of recent events such as war or natural disaster. For example, Dr Sivayokan (2011), a psychiatrist in Northern Sri Lanka, found that many new words and phrases had come into use to express emotional distress since the civil conflict in the area; and that 'a comprehensive understanding of these idioms would help in exploring the well-being and mental health of these communities' (p. 65).

Table 10.2 Ground rules for development

Local not global thinking
Based primarily on local knowledge
Individual and community rights prioritized
Culturally consistent
Ethical
Sustainable
Community based
Bottom-up
Home-grown
Avoiding mistakes in the North

It is important that agencies and individuals planning development take time to find out what the people concerned normally do about mental health problems and what services local people choose to access for help when suffering distress, with some idea of why they do so For example, what happens in Sri Lanka is that most rural people, and many city dwellers too, access a variety of sources of help for mental health problems, including indigenous healers and/or religious healing and of course support from family and community (see an example of the variety of healing accessed in a region of Sri Lanka see Table 4.1 in Chapter 4). Further, most people take a pragmatic approach making choices on the basis of affordability, ease of access and hearsay; the mental hospital (asylum) itself is often the last resort. Non-governmental agencies (NGOs) play some part in providing mental health and social care but sometimes their approaches are determined by western funding agencies rather than local needs, although usually by a mixture of the two. Something recently noted in Sri Lanka is that some types of indigenous spiritual healing, although preferred by local people to any other, are becoming very expensive because of rising costs of organizing them (Perera, 2013, personal communication). Consequently, psychiatric drug therapies, although popularly considered less effective and less desirable, are being increasingly accessed merely because they are cheap, being available free in government hospitals. In such a situation, development would need to enable people to access services they value; issues such as government policy on what is available in its hospitals and the more general one of affordability have to be faced.

Prioritizing local knowledge does not mean that information on what happens in HICs is ignored, but the limitations of western models and systems must be carefully assessed for local applicability and dangers sometimes implicit in merely copying western systems taken on board. Learning from mistakes in the North is considered later in this chapter.

Human rights

Perhaps asylums should never have been introduced in LMICs, but many still function in these countries and require urgent attention, not least to prevent violations of individual human rights. Excessive use of ECT as treatment and seclusion (solitary confinement) as a way of controlling patients in mental hospitals are well known and practices that are prevalent in many countries. However, in many LMICs, these practices are often free of regulation. Human rights should be at the top of the agenda when any new development is being planned and these should be interpreted in terms of both individual rights and community rights (Chapter 1). It is essential that there should be clear guidance and regulation of potentially harmful practices in hospitals; and the recognition of the right of local communities to have a say in conditions in hospitals and to have a voice in planning and development (see below). Also, adherence to community rights means that mental health development must be consistent with local cultural patterns and social conditions in the societies concerned.

In the field of international politics involving North–South interactions, humanitarian impulses are sometimes quoted as the reason for political, or even military, intervention in LMICs by some western countries (Bricmont, 2007). In similar vein, I have sometimes heard theargument by people advocating 'scaling up' mental health services in the Global South to the standards available in the Global North (see Chapter 8 for discussion of 'scaling up') that non-western populations have a 'human right' to have access to psychiatric treatment practised in the West—reminiscent of the nineteenth century claims by colonial powers about civilizing the natives. So care is needed in how the concept of 'human rights' is interpreted, cross-culturally and cross-nationally. In the field of mental health, I suggest that the notion of 'human rights' is limited to arguments for the rights of people to freedom, liberty and the exercise of personal choice; and great caution is needed if there are pressures to argue for alleged 'rights' to 'treatment' or even 'care', referring to models of what these mean in the West. A safeguard against this type of approach developing in a mental health system is to ensure that, whenever services are being developed, people who may use the services, or already have used them (both current service users and ex-service users), are involved in development and the regulation of services.

Cultural consistency, ethical and sustainable

The need for services to be consistent with the (cultural) norms of the society concerned is a ground rule that must be respected. The first thing to do when development is postulated is to clarify what people want from it and how they conceptualize good mental health and well-being. We see how major misunderstandings have arisen as a result of cultural differences when we look at the history of North–South interactions in the field of mental health over the past 100 years (discussed in many of the earlier chapters). Services that result from development must be acceptable to the people concerned and based primarily on local knowledge (for example, about mental health, idioms of distress and choice of people concerned) rather than being derived from imported knowledge, especially theories of health and illness and evidence of effectiveness derived in the West.

It is possible that overall service structures (such as in-patient units, rehabilitation units, and outreach services) used in the West may be adaptable for use worldwide but if they are copied, care should be taken to ensure that their detailed structures (for example, the organization of a hospital ward, the type of rehabilitation practised or the involvement of communities) are consistent with *local* cultural norms. Cultural consistency ties in with ethical development too. For development to be ethical, the services provided must be for the benefit of people of the country concerned regarded as 'self-defining *subjects*' rather than '*objects* of concern ... entitled to choose their way of life themselves' both as individuals and communities (Gasper, 2004, p. 195, italics in original). And sustainable development implies that what is developed will carry on into the future fitting into the mainstream of social and political structures without being dependent on ongoing input from other countries (as was the case in much of development in colonies). In the Global North, this may be achieved by regulations and laws usually related to general health services but in the Global South mental health and well-being services may be better 'looked after' by being linked (say) to religious organizations and/or local community groups or governmental systems.

Community based

Something that has become evident in discussions of mental health service development worldwide in a context of public health (Chapter 8) is the importance for discourse to focus on the communitarian 'social' dimension, rather than the individual 'biological'. So, services should focus more on dealing with people as communities as opposed to concentrating on individual ill-health, although both may be required. And there are questions around the meaning of 'community' and the sort of community-care that fits in to the (diverse) sociopolitical and cultural structures of societies in the Global South. In fact, not only are there wide differences between societies and communities in the rich North and (largely) poor South because of disparity of educational levels and wealth; but also the former, unlike the latter, tend to be predominantly 'western' in cultural background and outlook. All institution-based systems in the mental health field, whether asylums or newer systems such as outpatient clinics and day hospitals, tend to be basically similar whether located in the North or the South. But in the case of community care, it is absurd to think that a system suited to a society in the rich western North can usefully be replicated in the (poor) non-western South. Community care must be grounded in the societies that they are supposed to serve, with links with local people and agencies that are local. Unlike institutions, they have to be home-grown and developed bottom-up.

Avoid mistakes in the West

Serious doubts are currently being voiced about the effectiveness of mental health services based predominantly on bio-medical psychiatry in Britain (for example, Ramon and Williams, 2005; Tew, 2002), especially in the UK for ethnic minorities of Asian and African backgrounds (see Chapter 6 for discussions of these issues). They are still minority voices in terms of their power but increasingly persuasive as exemplified by articles in the *New York Review of Books* (Angell, 2011a,b) and *New York Times* (Frances, 2012). And today's minority opinion could well be established wisdom tomorrow. Like the asylum era, the current era of rigid diagnosis linked to early and prolonged medication may well be regretted in the Global North before too long. So care should be taken in developing services in the Global South not to enable easy access to psychotropic drugs and not to promote narrow, rigid systems of diagnosis. People and governments in the Global South need to be informed (and warned) of the experience in rich countries where now drug therapies dominate the mental health scene (Chapters 2 and 3) and regulations may be required in LMICs to limit the availability of some types of medication.

Summary

A basic principle of development is that we have to start by looking at what happens currently, locally, and work from there. Thinking locally is important to ensure social and cultural relevance of services and ownership by the people responsible for sustaining the results of development and also for cost-effectiveness. In most LMICs a variety of services are accessed by people, but usually only if they can afford to do so. The issue of funding is difficult and contentious. There is a role for foreign agencies, if only in kick-starting with funding and by demonstrating what happens in HICs that local people may wish to learn from. But it is important that they not impose models of care that local people find culturally alien or models that may be discarded in the West before long anyway, such as the narrow, diagnosis-based, bio-medical system of psychiatry.

The (incorrect) assumption that there is a common language of psychiatry and psychology that is universal or global, and that terms such as 'mental health' and 'mind' are given the same meaning across the world in all languages and cultures, seems to underpin the approach of MGMH and to some extent affects the more recent publications of WHO advocating in effect the imposition of evidence-based remedies of psychiatry for mental illness as defined in DSM and ICD (Chapter 8). Developing mental health in LMICs is not a simple matter of applying systems backed by 'evidence' from the West and approved by the dominant classes of both regions with (at most) minor tweaking for 'cultural sensitivity' and language translation. Established strategies commonly used in HICs are unlikely to be successful in LMICs where current conditions, cultural norms and past history are all very different to those in the Global North. In these circumstances, mental health and well-being development in terms of providing services in LMICs must be *homegrown*. Clearly, western help is needed and should be welcomed, but care should be taken to avoid the danger inherent in such help that it may impose western ideologies leading to popularizing drugs as the solution to social problems and opening the doors to developing markets for products from the Global North (see the following section).

North–South collaboration

In Chapter 2, I discussed the various traditions worldwide concerning mental health and illness. Yet, we need to face up to global interdependence of the nations of the world and that no one nation can go it alone in any field—not for long anyway and not very far. So in considering development in the Global South, there has to be a place for input from the Global North (developed countries) and vice versa. Interchange of knowledge both at theoretical and practical levels is to the advantage of both sides—cultures may be different but yet there are points of overlap, similarity and cultural hybridity. For example, it is noted earlier that 'collective trauma' may characterize the effects on mental health of people exposed to conflict and disaster in the non-western settings; but the concept of collective trauma after disasters was first mentioned by Erickson (1994), an American who had studied the aftermath of a natural disaster in the USA to describe the collective trauma reflected in 'a blow to basic tissues of social life that damages the bonds attaching people together [in a community]' (pp. 229–33). In other words, even some notions that seem almost culture-specific (in this case collective trauma) are not necessarily so and there is much that everyone can learn from North–South interchange (see below).

In planning transnational collaboration I suggest we should look to interchange of knowledge, ideas and practical strategies on equal terms based on respect and cross-cultural understanding: This must be on a level playing field or nearly so, and there is no place for the patronizing arrogance inherent in some western institutional practices that may have carried over from colonial times, nor for the 'colonial condition' among people in the South (see Chapters 5 and 7) that (in the context of development) results in disparaging the indigenous and imitating the 'western'. This means that for proper collaboration between North and South: (a) There is interchange of knowledge about mental health, forms of healing and medical systems; experts *travel both ways* not just West to East/North to South; and 'centres of excellence' holding s knowledge give equal status to both western and non-western knowledge. (b) Research around mental health is pursued on a broad front encompassing a broad range of activities around social science and various types of psychology including those embedded in religions, and community development models. Also, there is a need for action research into service-user involvement and innovations in amalgamation of religious healing and psychotherapy (Chapter 9). (c) It is acknowledged that psychiatry as practised in Euro-America is not universally applicable, that illness categories for mental health listed in DSM and ICD (see Chapter 6) mean very little outside Euro-America and in fact may merely mislead development aims; and mental health is to do with people's lives and experiences and not only about happenings inside the head—a matter of fundamental nlearning for psychiatrists to endure if they are to be involved in development.

Community development

The search for ways of improving well-being (and hence mental health) of people in LMICs is being pursued today in community projects and programmes initiated within many countries. Many of these programmes are not written up and seldom reported in international journals. They are conducted by small groups of people often under adverse conditions and severely under-resourced. Gathering together the knowledge and expertise inherent in these programmes could be an important prelude to mental health development. Some have come together as part of the worldwide movements under the overall category of 'service user and survivor networks', mostly functioning outside the official field of healthcare/health services. But there are many other stakeholders too that may have contributions to make. Essentially, community development is about involving people at grass roots from the start. The Global Health (TGH) Program (Weerackody and Fernando, 2011) proposed a process involving three overlapping stages for developing community mental health services in a LMIC that had recently emerged from armed conflict and a series of natural disasters, including the 2004 Indian Ocean tsunami: (a) Dialogue and consultation with communities using participatory research methods; (b) capacity building of the various actors in the mental health and psychosocial scene in both the statutory and NGO sectors, namely psychiatrists, nurses, counsellors, social workers, community workers and volunteers; and (c) integration of the emerging community mental health system with wider systems of social development and public health, indigenous medical practitioners, healers and religious organizations. The exact nature of a system that develops through such a process will depend on the priorities and approaches identified by communities themselves; it is likely to be acceptable to the community concerned and address the needs as perceived by them. If the process is linked closely with a community facility—for example, a religious organization—its sustainability and ownership by the community concerned could be ensured (p. 134).

Social determinants of health

Chapter 8 refers to the WHO document *Closing the gap in a generation: Health equity through action on the social determinants of health* (CSDH, 2008), and the book *The Spirit Level* by Wilkinson and Picket (2010), both of highlight the fact that the main (social) causes of all health problems (including 'mental' ill-health) centre on inequality, both across nations and within nations. Three types of action were proposed for addressing social determinants of health in the WHO document: Improving daily living conditions; tackling inequitable distribution of power, money and resources; and measuring and understanding the problem and assessing the impact of action. If mental health development in LMICs means anything at all, the most important way forward is clearly to address positively the causes of the social determinants of health through public policies. The challenges here are firmly with the politicians but pressure from organizations such as WHO on governments and international bodies such as the World Bank and International Monetary Fund could help greatly.

Bambra *et al.* (2005) pointed out nearly ten years ago the need for a 'mainstream debate about the ways in which the politics, power and ideology, which underpin it [social determinants of health] influence people's health' (Bambra *et al.*, 2005, p. 187). We are still waiting for this debate. The block at international level (explored a little in Chapter 8) may partly stem from reluctance of the West to risk jeopardizing its political and economic hold on the Global South. Policy change at a political level (say) to overcome—or even reduce—poverty may well be the most important way of promoting mental health in LMICs. It is essential that countries in the Global South, either individually or collectively, address the issues that result in (what have been identified as) social determinants of health. This should be the primary approach top-down in mental health development in LMICs.

Regulation of systems

As part of the top-down approach in development, regulation of some of the systems already in place and administrative action to prevent practices that counteract policies and programmes that promote community care may be necessary in some countries, especially those undergoing rapid economic change. At the top of the list is action to prevent gross abuse of individual human rights in places where people deemed to suffer from mental illness are housed, whether given diagnoses or not. Undoubtedly, these should apply to all hospitals and asylums but also to similar places run by religious organizations and other non-health organizations, and indeed to residencies of various sorts. Another area that requires regulation fairly urgently is that of activities of big business, especially the pharmaceutical industry. The anecdotes in Chapter 8 indicate the subtle ways in which the pharmaceutical industry may build its markets for selling neuroleptics, so regulation to prevent such activity may be difficult to enforce. Also, increasing regulation of markets may go against the current political policies of de-regulation of business activities because of neo-liberal policies (see Chapter 8) and so opposed by powerful western countries, or their effectiveness undermined through economic pressures. However, it is important to recognize that the social end result of the lack of regulation can be seriously detrimental to mental health development and to programmes that focus on community care. According to Bhargavi Davar (2012), since the easing of regulations (in about 2002) on starting private asylums in India, over 400 private asylums have been built in the country. But even if asylum development itself can be prevented, big business may penetrate the mental health field through public private partnerships (PPP) (discussed briefly in Chapter 8); and this too would need regulation. In countries where regulation is difficult to enforce, the answer may be to ban all for-profit business involvement in mental health development at least for the time being.

Conclusions

Plans for improving mental health and well-being in LMICs should be both top-down and bottom-up (Table 10.3). The main approach top-down should be based on addressing social determinants of health, preventing human rights violations in institutions and other places where people deemed mentally ill reside, running down where necessary systems (such as old-fashioned asylums) that date to colonial times, and protecting vulnerable communities from exploitation by big business interests. This last problem may be difficult to tackle and the simpler option may be to limit by law the involvement of big business in the mental health field and keep close watch on expenditure of Big Pharma in the field of mental health.

Models for bottom-up improvement should be basically community-based, rights-based and ethical in being clearly for the benefit of the people concerned and involving them in decision-making. Therefore, programmes should be developed in consultation with communities concerned and stakeholders in the community. The exact composition of stakeholders involved and the problems that need to be addressed would vary from country to country, encompassing local situations and cultures. Community development approaches may be the best but other similar ways of involving communities may well be preferred—and more acceptable politically—in some places. The

Table 10.3 Plans for development

Top-down development
Address social determinants of health
Regulate and run down where necessary current systems
Protect vulnerable communities from exploitation
Bottom-up development
Community based, rights based and ethical
In consultation with local communities and variety of stakeholders
Outcomes that are sustainable

outcomes are likely to vary from place to place; one model just cannot fit all. Information on what exactly is developed (for example, the use of different forms of treatment) can be drawn from far and wide and so there is space for North–South collaboration in an ethical framework (see above under North–South collaboration). Ideally the *local* mental health systems that is developed in a particular place must have the capacity for sustainability by being incorporated into the appropriate local political and social systems which may or may not be medical (in the way mental health systems are 'medical' in the Global North).

In short, the way for mental health and well-being development in LMICs lies in a two-pronged approach. A largely top-down approach (basically led politically) that addresses social determinants of health and regulation of services; and a bottom-up approach whereby services are developed in a process that is ethical and results in services that are sustainable and geared to social, psychological and cultural needs of the people concerned. Raising the funds necessary for building up these bottom-up services is a complicated matter. Clearly it would be necessary to shop around (mainly in HICs) with support of international bodies like WHO and World Bank. Some minor compromises may be required to suit their demands but it is essential in terms of long-term safety of people in LMICs that that the main guidelines discussed under 'ground rules' (above) are adhered to.

It is important that governments and NGOs involved in development in the Global South are aware of realities of development work in LMICs. Ground realities to consider in planning mental health and well-being services are summarized in Table 10.1. Ground rules that should be followed are listed in Table 10.2. The process that is most likely to yield best results is given in very broad outline in Table 10.3. The services that come about are not easy to forecast because essentially the development process is one that is dynamic and open-ended. The bottom-up (community development) approach in developing services on the ground may well result in a mixture of (a) schemes to support traditional indigenous systems adapting variations of traditional western systems; (b) or (more likely) breaking new ground by amalgamating what is locally available (but needs developing) with what local people consider is best from other countries; and (c) even more likely, local innovations in mixtures of social, religious and medical approaches.

11
Afterthoughts: Power, Diagnosis and the Majority World

As I was completing this book, the newest version (fifth edition) of the *Diagnostic and Statistical Manual of Mental Disorders* (DSM- 5) (APA, 2013) was published. The opposition to DSM 5 raised the question for the general public: '[D]oes mental illness really exist' (Doward, 2013, p. 1)? And the (British) Division of Clinical Psychology (part of the British Psychological Association—BPS) issued a position statement on psychiatric nosology calling for a change of paradigm in thinking about the Euro-American system of psychiatric diagnosis (DCP, 2013). Although, strictly speaking, DSM merely provides a system of categorization devised in the USA for the USA, its main use being as a reference for insurance companies paying practitioners for providing psychiatric and psychological treatment. This massive volume is recognized now as exercising power across the world in propagating western psychiatry: '[T]he political dominance of the US means that, as soon as a mental disorder is named in the DSM, that disorder becomes valid in the eyes of the many' (Burns, 2013, p. 1).

Chapter 8 explored the marketing of diagnosis that goes with the sale of drugs as remedies; but even more than psychiatric power linked to that of the pharmaceutical industry, the direction that development takes often comes from economic forces and aspects of geopolitical power. The thrust in Chapter 10 is that people in the Global South should develop something different to the sort of mental health services (based on Euro-American psychiatry) currently available in the Global North; and Chapter 9 suggests changes in mental health services that would benefit people in the Global North, even without abandoning psychiatric nosology altogether. So, two questions struck me as afterthoughts: First, where is psychiatry going to stand worldwide in the future? And second, how would the mass of people in the Global South, who today suffer from high levels of social suffering (to say the least), really fare vis-à-vis mental health and well-being?

Psychiatry

Since this book has talked a lot about the way psychiatry has played out over the years (mainly) in the Global North and now seriously penetrating the South, the question about its future status is relevant. In my view, it all depends on what happens to psychiatry in its bastion Euro-America, where it is currently in a state of crisis (Chapter 6). It is just possible that a type of psychiatry would emerge there that can have a useful role in the Global South. If such a 'world psychiatry' ever emerges, it will have to be something flexible, culturally sensitive and capable of being adapted for local conditions and cultures in different parts of the world. As in the case of systems of mental health, it would have to get integrated and grow bottom-up within each sociocultural setting, informed by a range of medical and healing systems that a professional 'world psychiatrist' can straddle. I do not see at present what that sort of psychiatry would be like, but its basis may well be reflected in the changes that are suggested in a recent special article in the *British Journal of Psychiatry* by Bracken *et al.* (2012):

> We [psychiatrists] need to develop an approach to mental health problems that is genuinely sensitive to the complex interplay of forces (biological, psychological, social and cultural) that underlie them and that can be used therapeutically. The evidence is becoming clear that to improve outcomes for our patients, we must focus more on contexts, relationships and the creation of services where the promotion of dignity, respect, meaning and engagement are prioritised. We must become more comfortable with cultural diversity, service user empowerment and the importance of peer support. (p. 432)

If psychiatry fails to adapt to the modern culturally diverse world over the next few years, the outlook is bleak for both the profession and mental health development in general. A narrow bio-medical psychiatry will then either become a mere adjunct to neurology, thereby losing the contribution it could make as a discipline that is potentially able to bring together within a medical framework social, psychological and biological dimensions of human beings, or it will lose its identity altogether within allopathic medicine. Its role as an adjunct of neurology would, in the Global South (where indigenous systems of medicine are likely to continue as a part of a plurality of medical systems), become merely a front for the pharmaceutical industry possibly linked to health conglomerates and MNCs. However, if psychiatry undergoes the sort of paradigm change envisaged by Bracken *et al.* (2012), its practice may become sufficiently flexible to play a constructive role in mental health systems worldwide.

Global power and voices of the poor

While suggesting a process of gradual development of mental health and well-being systems (or services) in the Global South (ideally in processes described in Chapter 10), I can see that development is unlikely to occur in a systematic way. At one extreme, if global power-politics of the future plays out in the way it seems to do today (Chapter 8), my suggested outline plan for development (in Chapter 10) may be no more than a vision and may well be just a dream. But what is more likely is that bits and pieces of development following various models will occur as opportunities arise and political will prevails. This is how development always happens and this is how things worked out in the Global North over the past 100 years. The fear is that the mechanics of global power would drive policies and projects in ways that satisfy mainly economic interests. If at least the ground rules, outlined in Chapter 10, are not taken on board, the chances are that market forces in a context of neo-liberalism (Chapter 8), perhaps even backed by an aggressive psychiatry allied with Big Pharma, will allow the spread of unadulterated bio-medical psychiatry to dominate the scene in the Global South, with perhaps a few pockets of independent action where these forces are resisted.

Chapter 10 calls for ethical standards in development of mental health services in LMICs, mostly countries where, compared to the Global North, the vast majority of people are poor and voiceless and remain culturally 'non-western' in many ways, with very different ideas about what mental health means and very different needs and wants when compared to most people in the rich western countries. If Euro-American global power is allowed to suppress cultural forms in the Global South that relate to 'mental health' (as happened, for example, with the indigenous cultures of the First Nations of America) that would be a tragedy for the people of the countries concerned and shame on us all, especially those agencies and funders of mental health in the rich countries of the West. On the other hand, if Euro-American cultural hegemony gives way in the face of economic and political pressures, perhaps of not only the BRIC countries (Brazil, Russia, India and China) but also others, non-western cultural values (still seen in most circles, in a carryover from colonialism, as 'second-class' cultures) may play a greater role globally as suggested in the case of China in the book *When China Rules the World: The End of the Western World and the Birth of a New Global Order* (Jacques, 2012), and the global scene in mental health may well be very different.

Conclusions

Psychiatry and mental health systems have always been more political than social or medical. In the field of mental health and issues around developing services for people with mental health problems, the global importance of cultural differences is only recently being recognized as crucial; and the power exerted by geopolitical forces, including that of MNCs, especially the multinational pharmaceutical companies, is now an important factor in determining what happens. The future in terms of mental health services in both the developed North and the developing South (the Majority World) is uncertain. The assumption is that western systems based on bio-medical psychiatry would triumph worldwide (as Coca-Cola and McDonald's seem to be doing) but that may well not be the case in the long run as the influence of countries such as China become more important. Although a common perception is that globalization equals 'westernization' (King, 1995; Pieterse, 1995), it may well result in the opposite, at least in some spheres. Mental health worldwide may look very different in 30 or 40 years.

Bibliography

Aakster, C. W. (1986) 'Concepts in alternative medicine', *Social Science and Medicine*, 22(2), 265–73.

Ackner, B., Harris, A. and Oldham, A. J. (1957) 'Insulin treatment of schizophrenia; controlled study', *Lancet*, 2, 607–11.

Ae-Ngibise, K., Cooper, S., Adiibokah, E., Akpalu, B, Lund, C., Doku, V. and The MHAPP Research Programme Consortium (2010) ' "Whether you like it or not people with mental problems are going to go to them": A qualitative exploration into the widespread use of traditional and faith healers in the provision of mental health care in Ghana', *International Review of Psychiatry*, 22(6), 558–67.

Allon, R. (1971) 'Sex, race, socio-economic status, social mobility, and process-reactive ratings of schizophrenia', *Journal of Nervous and Mental Disease*, 153, 343–50.

Amarasingham, L. R. (1980) 'Movement among traditional healers in Sri Lanka; A case study of a Sinhalese patient', *Culture, Medicine and Psychiatry*, 4, 71–92.

Anderson, B. (1991) *Imagined Communities, Reflections on the Origin and Spread of Nationalism* (London and New York, Verso).

Angell, M. (2005) *The Truth About Drug Companies How they Deceive Us and What to do About it* (New York: Random House).

Angell, M. (2011a) 'The epidemic of mental illness: why?', *The New York Review of Books*, 23 June 2011.

Angell, M. (2011b) 'The illusions of psychiatry', *The New York Review of Books*, 14 July 2011.

Anon (1851) 'Startling facts from the census', *American Journal of Insanity*, 8(2), 153–5.

APA (American Psychiatric Association) (1952) *Mental Disorders: Diagnostic and Statistical Manual* (Washington DC: American Psychiatric Association Press).

APA (American Psychiatric Association) (1994) *Diagnostic and Statistical Manual of Mental Disorders. DSM-IV*, 4th edn. (Washington DC: APA).

APA (American Psychiatric Association) (2000) *Diagnostic and Statistical Manual of Mental Disorders: DSM-IV-TR*, 4th edn. (Washington DC: American Psychiatric Publishing).

APA (American Psychiatric Association) (2013) DSM 5. *Diagnostic and Statistical Manual of Mental Disorders*, 5th edn. (Washington DC: American Psychiatric Publishing).

Au, S. and Tang, R. (2009) 'Mental health services for Chinese people', in S. Fernando and F. Keating (eds.) *Mental Health in a Multi-Ethnic Society. A Multidisciplinary Handbook*, 2nd edn. (London and New York: Routledge) pp. 187–95.

Babcock, J. W. (1895) 'The colored insane', *Alienist and Neurologist*, 16, 423–47.

Bains, J. (2005) 'Race, culture and psychiatry: A history of transcultural psychiatry', *History of Psychiatry*, 16(2), 139–54.

Bairoch, P. (1981) 'The main trends in National Economic Disparities since the industrial revolution', in P. Bairoch and M. Levy-Leboyer (eds) *Disparities in Economic Development Since the Industrial Revolution* (London: Palgrave Macmillan) cited by Davis, 2001.

Baldwin, J. (1969) *The Fire Next Time* (Harmondsworth: Penguin).

Bambra, C., Fox, D. and Scott-Samuel, A. (2005) 'Towards a politics of health', *Health Promotion International*, 20(2), 187–93. Retrieved 10 May 2013 from: http://heapro.oxfordjournals.org/content/20/2/187.full#ref-33.

Barnes, M. and Berke, J. (1971) *Two Accounts of a Journey Through Madness* (London: MacGibbon and Kee).

Barzun, J. (2000) *From Dawn to Decadence 500 Years of Western Cultural Life 1500 to the Present* (New York: HarperCollins).

Basham, A. L. (1976) 'The practice of medicine in ancient and medieval India', in C. Leslie (ed) *Asian Medical Systems; A Comparative Study* (Berkely, CA and London: University of California Press) pp. 18–43.

Bass, E., Sommerfield, J. and Kurup, A. S. (2011) *Social Determinants Approaches to Public Health. From Concept to Practice* (Geneva: WHO).

Bateson, G., Jackson, D., Haley, J. and Weakland, J. (1956) 'Toward a theory of schizophrenia', *Behavioural Science*, 1, 251–64.

Bayer, R. (1981) *Homosexuality and American Psychiatry: The Politics of Diagnosis* (New York: Basic Books).

Bebbington, P. E. (1978) 'The epidemiology of depressive disorder', *Culture, Medicine and Psychiatry*, 2, 297–341.

Bemme, D. and D'souza, N. (2012) 'Global mental health and its discontents' *Somatosphere*. Retrieved 10 May 2013 from: http://somatosphere.net/2012/07/global-mental-health-and-its-discontents.html.

Bentall, R. P. (2010) *Doctoring the Mind. Why Psychiatric Treatments Fail* (London: Penguin Books).

Berinstain, V. (1998) *Mughal India: Splendours of the Peacock Throne* (London: Thames and Hudson).

Bhabha, H. (1991) 'Foreword', in F. Fanon *Black Skin White Masks*, trans. C. L. Markham, 2nd impression (London: Pluto Press) pp. vii–xxvi.

Bhabha, H. (1994) *The Location of Culture* (London: Routledge).

Bhui, K. (ed) (2002) *Racism and Mental Health. Prejudice and Suffering* (London: Jessica Kingsley).

Bhui, K. and Olajide, D. (1999) *Mental Health Service Provision for a Multi-cultural Society* (London: Saunders).

Bleuler, E. (1950) *Dementia Præcox or the Group of Schizophrenias*, trans. J. Zitkin (New York: International Universities Press). Originally published in 1911.

Bloch, S. and Reddaway, P. (1984) *The Shadows over World Psychiatry* (London: Gollancz).

Boyle, M. (2002) *Schizophrenia. A Scientific Delusion?* 2nd edn (London: Routledge).

Bracken, P., Thomas, P., Timimi, S., Asen, E. . . . and Yeomans, D. (2012) 'Psychiatry beyond the current paradigm', *British Journal of Psychiatry*, 201, 430–4.

Bricmont, J. (2007) *Humanitarian Imperialism. Using Human Rights to Sell War*, trans. D. Johnstone, 8th edn. (New York: Monthly Review Press).

Bright, T. (1586) *A Treatise of Melancholy* (London: Vautrolier).

Bromberg, W. and Simon, F. (1968) 'The "protest" psychosis. A special type of reactive psychosis', *Archives of General Psychiatry*, 19, 155–60.

Burns, C. (2013) 'Are mental illnesses, such as PMS and depression culturally determined?', *The Guardian*, Monday 20 May 2013. Retrieved on 23 May 2013 from: http://m.guardian.co.uk/science/blog/2013/may/20/mental-illnesses-depression-pms-culturally-determined.

Burton, R. (1806) *The Anatomy of Melancholy*, 11th edn. (London: Hodson). First published in 1621.

Bussard, S. (2012) 'The price for private funding of the World Health Organization', *Le Temps*. Retrieved 12 June 2013 from: http://www.worldcrunch.com/price-private-funding-world-health-organization/world-affairs/the-price-for-private-funding-of-the-world-health-organization/c1s3121/.

Bynum, W. F. Jr. (1981) 'Rationales for therapy in British psychiatry, 1780–1835', in A. Scull (ed) *Madhouses, Mad-Doctors and Madmen. The Social History of Psychiatry in the Victorian Era* (London: Athlone Press) pp. 35–57.

Campbell, C. and Burgess, R. (2012) 'The role of communities in advancing the goals of the movement for global mental health', *Transcultural Psychiatry*, 49(3–4), 379–395.

Capra, F. (1982) *The Turning Point. Science, Society, and the Rising Culture* (London: Wildwood House).

Carlat, D. (2010) *Unhinged: The Trouble With Psychiatry – A Doctor's Revelation About a Profession in Crisis* (New York: Free Press).

Carmichael, S. and Hamilton, C. V. (1967) *Black Power. The Politics of Liberation in America* (New York: Random House).

Carothers, J. C. (1951) 'Frontal lobe function and the African', *Journal of Mental Science*, 97, 12–48.

Carothers, J. C. (1953) *The African Mind in Health and Disease. A Study in Ethnopsychiatry*, WHO Monograph Series No. 17 (Geneva: World Health Organisation).

Carothers, J. C. (1972) *The Mind of Man in Africa* (London: Stacey).

Carstairs, G. M. (1973) 'Psychiatric problems of developing countries', *British Journal of Psychiatry*, 123(3), 271–7.

Carstairs, G. M. and Kapur, R. L. (1976) *The Great Universe of Kota; Stress, Change and Mental Disorder in an Indian Village* (Berkeley, CA and Los Angeles: University of California Press).

Cartwright, S. A. (1981) (1851) 'Report on the diseases and physical peculiarities of the Negro race', reprinted from *New Orleans Medical and Surgical Journal*, May 1851: 691–715 in A. C. Caplan, H. T. Engelhardt and J. J. McCartney (eds) *Concepts of Health and Disease* (Reading, MA: Addison-Wesley, 1981), pp. 305–25.

Chamberlin, J. (1978) *On Our Own. Patient Controlled Alternatives to the Mental Health System* (New York: Hawthorn Books).

Chambers, R. (1992) *Rural Appraisal: Rapid, Relaxed and Participatory, Institute of Development Studies (IDS)*, Discussion Paper 311 (Brighton, Sussex: IDS).

Chambers, R. (1997) *Whose Reality Counts? Putting the First Last* (London: ITDG Publishing).

Charlton, J. I. (2000) *Nothing About Us Without Us. Disability, Oppression and Empowerment* (Berkeley, CA and London: University of California Press).

Choudhry, Y. and Bakhsh, Q. (2009) 'Counselling and day care for South Asian people', in S. Fernando and F. Keating (eds) *Mental Health in a Multi-Ethnic Society. A Multidisciplinary Handbook* (London and New York: Routledge) pp. 196–204.

Clarke, J. J. (1997) *Oriental Enlightenment. The Encounter between Asian and Western Thought* (New York and Abington: Routledge).

Clifford, T. (1984) *Tibetan Buddhist Medicine and Psychiatry: The Diamond Healing* (York Beach, Main: Samuel Weiser).

Coburn, D. (2004) 'Beyond the income inequality hypothesis: Class, neo-liberalism, and health inequalities', *Social Science and Medicine*, 58, 41–58.

Cohen, P. (1999) *New Ethnicities, Old Racisms?* (London: Zed Books).

Collins, P. Y., Patel, V., Joestl, S. S., March, D., Insel, T. R. and Dar, A. (2011) 'Grand challenges in global mental health', *Nature*, 475, 27–30.

Cooper, D. (1970) *Psychiatry and Anti-Psychiatry* (London: Paladin).

Cooper, J. and, Sartorius, N. (1977) 'Cultural and temporal variations in schizophrenia: A speculation on the importance of industrialization', *British Journal of Psychiatry*, 130(1), 50–5.

Cooper, J. E., Kendell, R. E., Gurland, B. J., Sharpe, L., Copeland, J. R. M. and Simon, R. (1972) *Psychiatric Diagnosis in New York and London*, Maudsley Monograph No. 20 (London: Oxford University Press).

Cox, J. (ed.) (1986) *Transcultural Psychiatry* (London: Croom Helm).

Craddock, N., Antebi, D., Attenburrow, M.-J. ... and Zammit, S. (2008) 'Wake-up call for British psychiatry', *British Journal of Psychiatry*, 193, 6–9.

Crane, R. (2009) *Mindfulness-Based Cognitive Therapy* (London and New York: Routledge).

CSDH (Commission on Social Determinants of Health) (2008) *Closing the gap in a generation: Health equity through action on the social determinants of health.* Final Report of the Commission on Social Determinants of Health (Geneva, World Health Organization). Retrieved 18 March 2013 from: http://www.who.int/social_determinants/thecommission/finalreport/en

Dalal, F. (1988) 'The racism of Jung', *Race and Class*, 29(3), 1–22.

Das, A. and Rao, M. (2012) 'Universal mental health: Re-evaluating the call for global mental health', *Critical Public Health*, 22(4), 183–9.

Davar, B. (2012) 'Legal frameworks for and against people with psychosocial disabilities', *Economic and Political Weekly*, XLVII(52), 123–31.

David, A. and Sartorius, N. (2013) 'Has psychiatric diagnosis labelled rather than enabled patients?', Head to Head Maudsley Debate. *British Medical Journal*, 347, 20–21.

Davidson, B. (1984) *Africa in History. Themes and Outlines* revised updated edn. (London: Paladin Books).

Davidson, L., Rakfeldt, J. and Strauss, J. (eds.) (2010) *The Roots of the Recovery Movement in Psychiatry. Lessons Learned* (Chichester, UK: Wiley-Blackwell).

Davis, M. (2001) *Late Victorian Holocausts. El Niño Famines and the Making of the Third World* (London and New York: Verso).

DCP (Division of Clinical Psychology) (2013) *Time for a Paradigm Shift*. Division of Clinical Psychology Position Statement on the Classification of Behaviour and Experience in Relation to Functional Psychiatric Diagnoses. Retrieved 15 July 2013 from: http://www.madinamerica.com/wp-content/uploads/2013/05/DCP-Position-Statement-on-Classification.pdf

Delay, J., Deniker, P. and Hart, J. M. (1952) 'Utilisation en thérapeutique psychiatrique d'une phenothiazine d'action centrale élective (4560 RP)', *Annals of Medical Psychology* (Paris), 110, 112–7. Cited by Moncrieff, 2009.

Demerath, N. J. (1942) 'Schizophrenia among primitives', *American Journal of Psychiatry*, 98, 703–07.

Devereux, G. (1939) 'Mohave culture and personality', *Character and Personality*, 8, 91–109.

Diener, E. (1984) 'Subjective well-being', *Psychological Bulletin*, 96, 542–75.

Diener, E. and Suh, E. M. (2000) 'Measuring subjective well-being to compare quality of life of cultures', in E. Diener and E. M. Suh (eds) *Culture and Subjective Well-being* (Cambridge, MA and London: MIT Press) pp. 3–12.

DOH (Department of Health) (1999) *National Service Framework for Mental Health. Modern Standards and Service Models* (London: DOH).

DOH (Department of Health) (2005) *Delivering Race Equality in Mental Health Care An Action Plan for Reform Inside and Outside Services and The Government's Response to the Independent Inquiry into the Death of David Bennett* (London: DOH).

Dols, M. W. (1992) *Majnūn: The Madman in Medieval Islamic Society* D. E. Immisch (ed) (Oxford: Clarendon Press).

Donald, A. (2001) 'The wal-marting of American psychiatry: An ethnography of psychiatric practice in the late twentieth century', *Culture, Medicine and Psychiatry*, 25(4), 427–39.

Doward, J. (2013) Medicine's new battleground: Does mental illness really exist?', *The Guardian*, 12 May 2013. Retrieved on 23 May 2013 from: http://m.guardian.co.uk/society/2013/may/12/medicine-dsm5-row-does-mental-illness-exist.

Dube, K.C. (1970) 'A study of prevalence and biosocial variables in mental illness in a rural and an urban community in Uttar Pradesh – India', *Acta Psychiatrica Scandinavica*, 46(4), 327–59.

Eagleton, T. (2000) *The Idea of Culture* (Oxford: Blackwell).

Easterly, W. (2006) *The White Man's Burden. Why the West's Efforts to Aid the Rest Have Done So Much Ill and So Little Good* (Oxford and New York: Oxford University Press).

Eisenberg, L. (2000) 'Is psychiatry more mindful or brainier than it was a decade ago?', *British Journal of Psychiatry*, 176, 1–5.

Elnagar, M. N., Maitra, P. and Rao, M. N. (1971) 'Mental health in an Indian rural community', *British Journal of Psychiatry*, 118, 499–503.

Engel, G. L. (1977) 'The need for a new medical model: A challenge for biomedicine', *Science*, 196(4286), 129–36.

Erickson, K. (1994) *A New Species of Trouble. The Human Experience of Disasters* (New York and London: Norton).

Ernst, W. (2010) *Mad Tales from the Raj: Colonial Psychiatry in South Asia 1800–1858* (London and New York: Anthem Press).

Esteva, G. and Prakash, M. (1977) 'From global thinking to local thinking', in M. Rahnema and V. Bawtree (eds) *The Post-Development Reader* (London and New Jersey: Zed Books) pp. 277–89.

Evarts, A. B. (1913) 'Dementia precox in the colored race', *Psychoanalytic Review*, 14, 388–403.

Eze, E. (1997) (ed.) *Race and the Enlightenment. A Reader* (Cambridge, MA: Blackwell).

Fabrega, H. (2009) *History of Mental Illness in India. A Cultural Psychiatry Retrospective* (Delhi: Motilal Banarsidass).

Fanon, F. (1952) *Peau Noire, Masques Blancs* (Paris: Editions de Seuil), trans. C. L. Markmann, *Black Skin, White Masks* (New York: Grove Press, 1967).

Fanon, F. (1959) *L'An Cinq, de la Révolution Algérienne.* (Paris: Maspero), trans. H. Chevalier, *A Dying Colonialism* (New York: Grove Press 1965).

Fanon, F. (1961) *Les Damnés de la terre.* (Paris: Francois Maspero), trans. C. Farrington, *The Wretched of the Earth* (Harmondsworth: Penguin 1967).

Fanon, F. (1965) *A Dying Colonialism* trans. by H. Chevalier (New York: Grove Press).

Fanon, F. (1967) *The Wretched of the Earth,* trans. by C. Farrington (Harmondsworth: Penguin).

Faris, R. E. L. (1967) *Mental Disorders in Urban Areas* (Chicago: University of Chicago Press).

Faris, R. E. L. and Dunham, H. W. (1939) *Mental Disorders in Urban Areas: An Ecological Study of Schizophrenia and Other Psychoses* (Chicago: University of Chicago Press).

Faulkner, A. and Thomas, P. (2002) 'User-led research and evidence-based medicine', *British Journal of Psychiatry*, 180(1), 1–3.

Featherstone, M. and Lash, S. (1995) 'Globalization, modernity and the spatialization of social theory: An introducton', in M. Featherstone, S. Lash and R. Robertson (eds) *Global Modernities* (London and New Delhi: Sage) pp. 1–24.

Felix, R. H. and Bowers, R. V. (1948) 'Mental hygiene and socio-environmental factors', *Millbank Fund Quarterly*, 26, 125.

Fennell, M. V. (2009) 'Cognitive behaviour therapy for depressive disorders', in M. G. Gelder, N. C. Andreasen, J. J. López-Ibor Jr and J. R. Geddes (eds) *New Oxford Textbook of Psychiatry*, 2nd edn., vol 2 (Oxford: Oxford University Press) pp. 1304–13.

Fernando, S. (1988) *Race and Culture in Psychiatry* (London: Croom Helm). Reprinted as paperback Routledge, London 1989.

Fernando, S. (1991) *Mental Health, Race and Culture* (London: Macmillan–Mind).

Fernando, S. (1995) (ed.) (2009) *Mental Health in a Multi-Ethnic Society. A Multi-Disciplinary Handbook*, 2nd edn. (London and New York. Routledge).

Fernando, S. (2002) *Mental Health, Race and Culture*, 2nd edn. (Basingstoke: Palgrave).

Fernando, S. (2003) *Cultural Diversity, Mental Health and Psychiatry. The Struggle against Racism* (Hove, East Sussex and New York: Brunner-Routledge).

Fernando, S. (2005) 'Multicultural mental health services: Projects for minority ethnic communities in England', *Transcultural Psychiatry*, 42(3), 420–36.

Fernando, S. (2009) 'Inequalities and the politics of "race" ', in S. Fernando and F. Keating (eds) *Mental Health in a Multi-Ethnic Society*, 2nd edn. (London: Routledge) pp. 42–57.

Fernando, S. (2010) *Mental Health, Race and Culture*, 3rd edn. (Basingstoke and New York: Palgrave).

Fernando, S. (2011) 'A "global" mental health program or markets or Big Pharma?', *Openmind*, 168, 22.

Fernando, S. and Keating, F. (2009a) *Mental Health in a Multi-ethnic Society. A Multi-Disciplinary Handbook,* 2nd edn. (London and New York: Routledge).

Fernando, S. and Keating, F. (2009b) 'The way ahead', in S. Fernando and F. Keating (eds) *Mental Health in a Multi-Ethnic Society. A Multi-Disciplinary Handbook,* 2nd edn. (London and New York: Routledge) pp. 235–58.

Fernando, S. and Weerackody, C. (2009) 'Challenges in developing community mental health services in Sri Lanka', *Journal of Health Management,* 11(1), 195–208.

Fernando, S., Ndegwa, D. and Wilson, M. (1998) *Forensic Psychiatry, Race and Culture* (London: Routledge).

Fernando, S., Trivedi, P. and Ferns, P. (2013) 'Recovery and well-being', in K. Bhui (ed) *Elements of Culture and Mental Health. Clinical Questions for Clinicians* (London: RCPsych Publications).

Ferns, P. (2009) 'The challenges of race equality and cultural capability (RECC) training', in S. Fernando and F. Keating (eds) *Mental Health in a Multi-Ethnic Society. A Multidisciplinary Handbook,* 2nd edn. (London and New York: Routledge) pp. 108–21.

Field, M. J. (1958) 'Mental disorder in rural Ghana', *Journal of Mental Science,* 104, 1043–51.

Field, M. J. (1960) *Search for Security: An Ethnocentric Study of Rural Ghana* (Evanston, Ill.: Northwestern University Press).

Foucault, M. (1967) *Madness and Civilization. A History of Insanity in the Age of Reason* (London: Tavistock). Originally published in French as *Histoire de la Folie* (Paris: Libraire Plon) 1961.

Foucault, M. (2006) *History of Madness,* ed. Jean Khalfa, trans. Jonathan Murphy and Jean Khalfa (London and New York: Routledge).

Frances, A. (2012) 'Diagnosing the D. S. M', *New York Times* 12 May 2012, p. A19. Retrieved 31 May 2012 from: http://www.nytimes.com/2012/05/12/opinion/break-up-the-psychiatric-monopoly.html?_r=1&emc=eta1.

Freud, S. (1913) *Totem and Taboo* (Vienna: Hugo Heller) trans. and pub. in English (London: Routledge and Kegan Paul) 1950.

Friedman, J. (1995) 'Global system, globalization and the parameters of modernity', in M. Featherstone, S. Lash and R. Robertson (eds) *Global Modernities* (London and New Delhi: Sage) pp. 69–90.

Gaines, A. D. (ed.) (1992) *Ethnopsychiatry. The Cultural Construction of Professional and Folk Psychiatries* (New York: State University of New York Press).

Galton, F. (1904) 'Eugenics: Its definition, scope, and aims', *American Journal of Sociology,* 10(1), 1–25.

Gamwell, L. and Tomes, N. (1995) *Madness in America. Cultural and Medical Perceptions of Mental Illness before 1914* (New York: Cornell University Press).

Gasper, D. (2004) *The Ethics of Development From Economism to Human Development* (Edinburgh: Edinburgh University Press).

Gates Foundation (2010) 'Global health strategy overview', *Bill and Melinda Gates Foundation.* Retrieved 10 May 2013 from: http://www.gatesfoundation.org/global-health/Documents/global-health-strategy-overview.pdf.

Gelfand, M. (1964) *Medicine and Custom in Africa* (Edinburgh and London: Livingstone).

Gilbert, P. (2007) 'The spiritual foundation: Awareness and context for people's lives today', in M. E. Coyte, P. Gilbert and V. Nicholls (eds) *Spirituality, Values and Mental Health* (London and Philadelphia: Jessica Kingsley) pp. 19–43.

Goldacre, B. (2012) *Bad Pharma How Drug Companies Mislead Doctors and Harm Patients* (London: Fourth Estate).

Gordon, H. L. (1934) 'The mental capacity of the East African native', *Journal of the African Society*, 33, 227.

Gosden, R. and Beder, S. (2001) 'Pharmaceutical industry agenda setting in mental health policies', *Ethical Human Sciences and Services*, 3(3), 147–59.

Graham, H. (1986) *The Human Face of Psychology. Humanistic Psychology in its Historical Social and Cultural Context* (Milton Keynes and Philadelphia: Open University Press).

Graham, T. F. (1967) *Medieval Minds Mental Health in the Middle Ages* (London: Allen & Unwin).

Green, E. M. (1914) 'Psychoses among Negroes – a comparative study', *Journal of Nervous and Mental Disorder*, 41, 697–708.

Gunaratne, B. H. (2002) *Mindfulness in Plain English* (Boston: MA: Wisdom Publications).

Gupta, M. (2007) 'Does evidence-based medicine apply to psychiatry?', *Theoretical Medicine and Bioethics*, 28(2), 103–20.

Hacker, A. (1992) *Two Nations Black and White, Separate, Hostile, Unequal* (New York: Charles Scribners).

Hacking, I. (1995) 'The looping effects of human kinds', in D. Sperber, D. Premark and A. J. Premark (eds) *Causal Cognition: A Multidisciplinary Approach* (Oxford: Oxford University Press) pp. 351–83.

Hacking I. (1999) *The Social Construction of What?* (Cambridge, MA and London: Harvard University Press).

Haig-Brown, C. (1988) *Resistance and Renewal. Surviving the Indian Residential School* (Vancouver: Arsenal Pulp Press).

Haley, J. (1963) *Strategies of Psychotherapy* (New York: Grune and Stratton).

Hall, S. (1992) 'New ethnicities', in J. Donald and A. Ratansi (eds) *'Race' Culture and Difference* (London: Sage) pp. 252–9.

Hall, S., Critcher, C., Jefferson, T., Clarke, J. and Roberts, B. (1978) *Policing the Crisis. Mugging, the State, and Law and Order* (London: MacMillan).

Halliburton, M. (2004) 'Finding a fit: Psychiatric pluralism in South India and its implications for WHO studies of mental disorder', *Transcultural Psychiatry*, 41(1), 80–9.

Hammer, L. (2000) *Dragon Rises, Red Bird Flies. Psychology, Energy and Chinese Medicine* (Barrytown, NY: Station Hill Press).

Harmer, A. (2012) Who's funding WHO?', *Global Health Policy*, Retrieved 12 June 2013 from http://www.globalhealthpolicy.net/?p=826.

Harrison, P. (1979) *Inside the Third World: The Anatomy of Poverty* (Harmondsworth: Penguin).

HEA (Health Education Authority) (1997) *Mental Health Promotion* (London: HEA).

Healy, D. (1990) *The Suspended Revolution. Psychiatry and Psychotherapy Re-examined* (London and Boston: Faber and Faber).

Healy, D. (2001) 'Evidence-based psychiatry?', *Psychiatric Bulletin*, 25, 290–91.

Higginbotham, N. and Marsella, A. J. (1988) 'International consultation and the homogenization of psychiatry in Southeast Asia', *Social Science and Medicine*, 27(5), 553–61.

Hobart, A. (2003) *Healing Performances of Bali: Between Darkness and Light* (New York and Oxford: Berghahn Books).

Holdcroft, L. E. (1978) *The Rise and Fall of Community Development in Developing Countries, 1950–1965,* MSU Rural Development Papers, Michigan State University, Paper no.2. Cited by MacDonald, 1992.

Hollingshead A. B. and Redlich, F. C. (1958) *Social Class and Mental Illness: A Community Study* (New York: Wiley).

Home Department (1999) *The Stephen Lawrence Inquiry. Report of an Inquiry by Sir William Macpherson of Cluny* (London: The Stationery Office).

Hopper, K. (1991). 'Some old questions for the new cross-cultural psychiatry', *Medical Anthropology Quarterly*, 5(4), 299–330.

Hopper, K. and Wanderling, J. (2000) 'Revisiting the developed versus developing country distinction in course and outcome in schizophrenia: Results from ISoS, the world collaborative follow up project', *Schizophrenia Bulletin*, 26(4), 835–46.

Horton R. (2007) 'Launching a new movement for mental health', *Lancet*, 370, 806.

Htwe, F. (2001) *Power in Medicine: British Imperialism and Health Provision in Burma, 1886–1936*. Research dissertation held at Wellcome Trust Foundation, London.

Hulme, D. (2007) *The Making of the Millennium Development Goals: Human Development Meets Results-based Management in an Imperfect World*. Working Paper 16 of the Brooks World Poverty Institute (BWPI) at University of Manchester (Manchester: BWPI). Retrieved 15 July 2013 from: http://www.bwpi.manchester.ac.uk/resources/Working-Papers/bwpi-wp-1607.pdf

IASC (Inter-Agency Standing Committee) (2007) *IASC Guidelines on Mental Health and Psychosocial Support in Emergency Settings* (Geneva: IASC) Retrieved on 15 July 2013 from: http://www.who.int/mental_health/emergencies/guidelines_iasc_mental_health_psychosocial_june_2007.pdf

Ingleby, D. (1980) *Critical Psychiatry. The Politics of Mental Health* (New York: Pantheon Books). Republished by Free Association Books, London 2004.

Ingleby, D. (1982) 'The Social construction of mental illness', in P. Wright and A. Treacher (eds) *The Problem of Medical Knowledge. Examining the Social Construction of Medicine* (Edinburgh: Edinburgh University Press) pp. 123–43.

Ingleby, D. (2014) (in press) 'Global mental health', in A. Scull (ed) *Cultural Sociology of Mental Illness. An A-Z Guide* (Thousand Oaks, CA: Sage Publications).

Inyama, C. (2009) 'Race relations, mental health and human rights – the legal framework', in S. Fernando and F. Keating (eds) *Mental Health in a Multi-Ethnic Society. A Multidisciplinary Handbook* (London and New York: Routledge) pp. 27– 41.

Jablensky, A., Schwarz, R. and Tomov, T. (1980) 'WHO collaborative study on impairments and disabilities associated with schizophrenic disorders', *Acta Psychiatrica Scandinavica*, 62, Suppl. 285, 152–63.

Jacob, K. S. (2011) 'Repackaging mental health programs in low- and middle-income countries', *Indian Journal of Psychiatry* 53(3), 195–8.

Jacques, M. (2012) *When China Rules The World*, 2nd edn. (London: Penguin Books).

Jain, S. and Jadhav, S. (2009) 'Pills that swallow policy: Clinical ethnography of a community mental health program in northern India', *Transcultural Psychiatry*, 46(1), 60–85.

Jaggi, O. P. (1981) *Ayurveda: Indian System of Medicine*, vol. 4, 2nd edn. (Delhi: Atma Ram).

Jarvis, E. (1852) 'On the supposed increase of insanity', *American Journal of Insanity*, 8, 333–64.

Jilek, W. G. (1982) *Indian Healing. Shamanistic Ceremonialism in the Pacific Northwest Today* (Surry BC and Blaine WA: Hancock House).

Johnstone, L. (2000) *Users and Abusers of Psychiatry. A Critical Look at Psychiatric Practice*, 2nd edn. (London and Philadelphia: Routledge).

Jones, J. (1983) *Community Development and Health Issues. A Review of Existing Theory and Practice* (Edinburgh: Community Projects Foundation) cited by MacDonald, 1992.

Jones, M. (1968) *Social Psychiatry in Practice* (Harmondsworth: Penguin).

Jones, J. and Hunter, D. (1995) 'Qualitative research: Consensus methods for medical and health services research', *British Medical Journal*, 311, 376–80.

Jung, C. G. (1930) 'Your negroid and Indian behaviour', *Forum*, 83(4), 193–9.

Jung, C. G. (1939) 'The dreamlike world of India', *Asia (New York)*, 39(1), 5–8, reprinted in H. Read, M. Fordham and G. Adler (eds) (1964) *Civilization in Transition. Collected Works of C. G. Jung* vol. 10 (London: Routledge and Kegan Paul) pp. 515–24.

Kakar, S. (1984) *Shamans, Mystics and Doctors: A Psychological Inquiry into India and its Healing Tradition* (London: Unwin Paperbacks).

Kalathil, J. (2007) *Recovery and Resilience: African, African-Caribbean and South Asian Women's Narratives of Recovering from Mental Distress* Report on findings from a research project carried out for Mental Health Foundation (MHF) (London: MHF).

Kapferer, B. (1991) *A Celebration of the Demons. Exorcism and the Aesthetics of Healing in Sri Lanka* (Oxford and Washington: Berg Publishers and Smithsonian Institute Press).

Kaptchuk, T. J. (2000) *Chinese Medicine the Web That Has No Weaver* (London: Rider).

Karenga, M. (1982) *Introduction to Black Studies* (Los Angeles: Kawaida Publications).

Karenga, M. and Carruthers, J. H. (1962) *Kemet and the African Worldview. Research, Rescue and Restoration* Part 3 (Los Angeles: University of Sankore Press).

Katz, M. M., Marsella, A., Dube, K. C., Olatawura, M., Takahashi, R., Nakane, Y., Wynne, L. C., Gift, T., Brennan, J., Sartorius, N. and Jablensky, A. (1988) 'On expression of psychosis in different cultures: Schizophrenia in an Indian and in a Nigerian community', *Culture, Medicine and Psychiatry*, 12, 331–55.

Keller, R. C. (2007a) *Colonial Madness. Psychiatry in French North Africa* (Chicago and London: University of Chicago Press).

Keller, R. C. (2007b) 'Taking science to the colonies: Psychiatric innovation in France and North Africa', in S. Mahone and M. Vaughan (eds) *Psychiatry and Empire* (Basingstoke: Palgrave Macmillan) pp. 17–40.

Kendell, R. E. and Jablensky, A. (2003) 'Distinguishing between the validity and utility of psychiatric diagnoses', *American Journal of Psychiatry*, 160(1), 4–12.

Khalfa, J. (2006) 'Introduction', in M. Foucault *History of Madness*, ed. J. Khalfa, trans. J. Murphy and J. Khalfa (London and New York: Routledge) pp. xiii–xxv.

Khan, M. M. (2006) 'Murky waters: The pharmaceutical industry and psychiatrists in developing countries', *Psychiatric Bulletin*, 30, 85–8.

Khin-Maung-Zaw (1997) 'Psychiatric services in Myanmar: A historical perspective', *Psychiatric Bulletin*, 21, 506–9.

Kickbusch, I. (2010) 'Health in all policies: The evolution of the concept of horizontal health governance', in I. Kickbusch and K. Buckett (eds) *Implementing Health in All Policies: Adelaide 2010* (Rundle Mall, South Australia: Department of Health) pp. 11–23.

Kiev, A. (1964) *Magic, Faith and Healing. Studies in Primitive Psychiatry Today* (New York: The Free Press of Glencoe).

King, A. D. (1995) 'The times and spaces of modernity (or who needs postmodernism?)', in M. Featherstone, S. Lash and R. Robertson (eds) *Global Modernities* (London and New Delhi: Sage) pp. 108–23.

Kirmayer, L. J. (1989) 'Cultural variations in the response to psychiatric disorders and emotional distress', *Social Science and Medicine*, 29(3), 327–39.

Kirmayer, L. J. (2006) 'Beyond the "new cross-cultural psychiatry": Cultural biology, discursive psychology and the ironies of globalisation', *Transcultural Psychiatry*, 43(1), 126–44.

Kirmayer, L. J. (2012) 'Cultural competence and evidence-based practice in mental health; Epistemic communities and the politics of pluralism', *Social Science and Medicine*, 75, 249–56.

Kirmayer, L., Groleau, D., Guzder, J., Blake, C. and Jarvis, E. (2003) 'Cultural consultation: A model for mental health services for multicultural societies', *Canadian Journal of Psychiatry*, 48(3), 145–53.

Kirsch, I. (2009) *The Emperor's New Drugs Exploding the Antidepressant Myth* (London: Bodley Head).

Kleinman, A. (1977) 'Depression, somatization and the "new cross cultural psychiatry"', *Social Science and Medicine*, 11, 3–10.

Kleinman, A. (1980) 'Major conceptual and research issues for cultural (anthropological) psychiatry', *Culture, Medicine and Psychiatry*, 4, 3–13.

Kleinman, A. (1995) *Writing at the Margin. Discourse between Anthropology and Medicine* (Berkeley CA and London: University of California Press).

Kleinman, A. and Good, B. (1985a) *Culture and Depression Studies in the Anthropology and Cross-Cultural Psychiatry of Affect and Disorder* (Berkeley CA: University of California Press).

Kleinman, A. and Good, B. (1985b) 'Introduction: Culture and depression', in A. Kleinman and B. Good (eds) *Culture and Depression. Studies in the Anthropology and Cross-Cultural Psychiatry of Affect and Disorder* (Berkley, CA and London: University of California Press) pp. 1–33.

Kloos, B. (2005) 'Creating new possibilities for promoting liberation, well-being, and recovery: Learning from experiences of psychiatric consumers/survivors', in G. Nelson and I Prilleltensky (eds) *Community Psychology: In Pursuit of Well-being and Liberation* (Basingstoke: Palgrave-Macmillan) pp. 426–47.

Kohrt, B. A. and Hruschka, D. J. (2010) 'Nepali concepts of psychological Trauma: The role of idioms of distress, ethnopsychology and ethnophysiology in alleviating suffering and preventing stigma', *Culture, Medicine and Psychiatry*, 34(2), 322–52.

Kraepelin, E. (1896) *Psychiatrie*. 5th edn (Leipzig: Verlag von Johann Ambrosius Barth).

Kraepelin, E. (1899) *Psychiatrie: ein Lehrbuch fur Studirende und Artze*, 6th edn. (Leipzig: Verlag von Johann Ambrosius Barth).

Kraepelin, E. (1913) *Manic Depressive Insanity and Paranoia*, trans. of *Lehrbuch der Psychiatrie* R. M. Barclay, 8th edn., vols 3 and 4 (Edinburgh: Livingstone).

Kraepelin, E. (1921) *Manic-Depressive Insanity and Paranoia*, trans. and ed. R. M. Barclay and G. M. Robertson (Edinburgh: Livingstone).

Kuhn, T. S. (1962) *The Structure of Scientific Revolutions*, 3rd edn. (Chicago and London: University of Chicago Press).

Kuhn, T. S. (2012) *The Structure of Scientific Revolutions*, 4th edn. (Chicago and London: University of Chicago Press).

Kumaranayake, L. and Walker, D. (2002) 'Cost-effectiveness analysis and priority-setting: Global approach without local meaning', in L. Kelley, K. Buse and S. Fustukian (eds) *Health Policy in a Globalising World* (Cambridge: Cambridge University Press) pp. 140–56.

Laing, R. D. (1967) *The Politics of Experience* (Harmondsworth: Penguin).

Laing, R. D. and Esterson, E. (1964) *Sanity, Madness and the Family* (London: Tavistock).

Lambo, A. (1964) 'Patterns of psychiatric care in developing African countries', in A. Kiev (ed) *Magic, Faith and Healing: Studies in Primitive Psychiatry Today*, Part 4 (New York: Free Press of Glencoe) pp. 443–53.

Lambo, A. (1969) 'Traditional African cultures and Western medicine', in F. N. L. Poynter (ed) *Medicine and Culture* (London: Wellcome Institute of the History of Medicine) pp. 201–10.

Last, M. and Chavunduka, G. L. (1986) (eds) *The Professionalisation of African Medicine* (Manchester: Manchester University Press).

Law, J. (2006) *Big Pharma. How the World's Biggest Drug Companies Control Illness* (London: Constable).

Law, T. (2011) *Psychiatry in Nigeria: How and why the field of psychiatry was exported to colonial Nigeria, how it evolved. And the problems it faced*, Thesis in Medical Sciences with History of Medicine. Available at Wellcome Trust Library, London.

Lawrence, P. (2003) 'Kāli in a context of terror. The tasks of a goddess in Sri Lanka's civil war', in R. F. McDermott and J. J. Kripal (eds) *Encountering Kāli. In the Margins, at the Centre, in the West* (Berkeley, CA, Los Angeles and London: University of California Press) pp. 100–79.

Leff, J. (1973) 'Culture and the differentiation of emotional states', *British Journal of Psychiatry*, 123, 299–306.

Leff, J. (1974) 'Transcultural influences on psychiatrists' rating of verbally expressed emotion', *British Journal of Psychiatry*, 125, 336–40.

Leff, J. (1975) '"Exotic" treatments and Western psychiatry', *Psychological Medicine*, 5, 125–28.

Leff, J. (1977) 'The cross-cultural study of emotions', *Culture, Medicine and Psychiatry*, 1, 317–50.

Leff, J. (1981) *Psychiatry Around the Globe* (New York: Dekker).

Leff, J. (1986) 'The epidemiology of mental illness across cultures', in J. L. Cox (ed) *Transcultural Psychiatry* (London: Croom Helm) pp. 23–36.

Leff, J., Wig, N. N., Bodi, H., Menon, D. K., Kuipers, L., Korten, A., Ernberg, G., Day, R., Sartorius, N. and Jablensky, A. (1990). 'Relatives' expressed emotion and the course of schizophrenia in Chandigarh', *British Journal of Psychiatry*, 156(3), 351–6.

Leighton, A. H. and Hughes, J. M. (1961) 'Cultures as causative of mental disorder', *Millbank Memorial Fund Quarterly*, 39(3), 446–70.

Leighton, A. H. Lambo, T. A., Hughes, C. C., Leighton, D. C., Murphy, J. M. and Macklin, D. M. (1963) *Psychiatric Disorder among the Yoruba* (New York: Cornell University Press).

Lewis, A. (1965) 'Chairman's opening remarks', in A. V. S. De Rueck and R. Porter (eds) *Transcultural Psychiatry. A Ciba Foundation Symposium* (London: J & A Churchill) pp. 1–3

Lexchin, J. (1992) 'Pharmaceutical promotion in the third world', *Journal of Drug Issues*, 22(2), 417–53.

Lindholm, C. (1996) *Islamic Middle East. An Historical Anthropology* (Oxford and Cambridge MA: Blackwell).

Linnett P. (1999) 'Thoughts on 'user involvement', *Openmind*, 98, 18–20.

Littlewood, R. and Lipsedge, M. (1982) *Aliens and Alienists: Ethnic Minorities and Psychiatry* (London: Penguin).

Littlewood, R. and Lipsedge, M. (1997) *Aliens and Alienists: Ethnic Minorities and Psychiatry*, 3rd edn. (London: Routledge).

LSHTM (London School of Hygiene and Tropical Medicine) (2013) 'Gift establishes nine new scholarships for global mental health' *LSHTM*. Retrieved on 10 May 2013 from: http://www.lshtm.ac.uk/newsevents/news/2013/nine_new_scholarships.html.

MacDonald, J. J. (1992) *Primary Health Care. Medicine in its Place* (London: Earthscan Publications).

Macey, D. (2000) *Frantz Fanon A Life* (London: Granta Books).

Maddison, A. (1998) *Chinese Economic Performance in the Long Run* (Paris: Organisation for Economic Co-operation and Development). Cited by Davis, 2001.

Mahone, S. (2007) 'East African psychiatry and the practical problems of empire', in S. Mahone and M. Vaughan (eds) *Psychiatry and Empire* (Basingstoke: Palgrave Macmillan).

Malik, R., Fateh, R. and Haque, R. (2009) 'The Marlborough cultural therapy centre', in S. Fernando and F. Keating (eds) *Mental Health in a Multi-Ethnic Society. A Multidisciplinary Handbook* (London and New York: Routledge) pp. 174–86.

Marx, K. (1978) 'The British rule in India', in R. C. Tucker (ed) *The Marx-Engels Reader*, 2nd edn. (New York: Norton) pp. 653–8.

Masood, E. (2009) *Science and Islam. A History* (London: Icon Books).

Maudsley, H. (1867) *The Physiology and Pathology of Mind* (New York: D. Appleton).

Maudsley, H. (1879) *The Pathology of Mind* (London: Macmillan).

Maziak, W. (2006) 'Health in the middle East', *British Medical Journal*, 333, 815–16.

Mbiti, J. S. (1989) *African Religions and Philosophy*, 2nd revised and enlarged edn. (Harlow, Essex: Heineman).

McClintock, A. (1995) *Imperial Leather. Race, Gender and Sexuality in the Colonial Contest* (New York and London: Routledge).

McCulloch, J. (1983) *Black Soul White Artefact. Fanon's Clinical Psychology and Social Theory* (Cambridge: Cambridge University Press).

McCulloch, J. (1995) *Colonial Psychiatry and 'The African Mind'* (Cambridge: Cambridge University Press).

McGovern, D. and Cope, R. (1987) 'The compulsory detention of males of different ethnic groups, with special reference to offender patients', *British Journal of Psychiatry*, 150, 505–12.

McInnes, C. and Lee, K. (2012) *Global Health and International Relations* (Cambridge and Malden, MA: Polity Press).

McQueen, D. V. (1978) 'The history of science and medicine as theoretical sources for the comparative study of contemporary medical systems', *Social Science and Medicine*, 12, 69–74.

Mental Capacity Act (Chapter 9) (2005) London: The Stationery Office. Retrieved 10 May 2013 from: http://www.legislation.gov.uk/ukpga/2005/9/contents

Mental Health Act (Chapter 12) (2007) London: The Stationery Office. Retrieved 10 May 2013 from: http://www.legislation.gov.uk/ukpga/2007/12/contents

Metzl, J. (2009) *The Protest Psychosis How Schizophrenia Became a Black Disease* (Boston MA: Beacon Press).

Mills, C. (2013) *Decolonizing Global Mental Health; The Psychiatrization of the Majority World* (London: Routledge) *in press*.

Mills, J. H. (2000) *Madness, Cannabis and Colonialism. The 'Native Only' Lunatic Asylums of British India 1857–1900* (Basingstoke: Macmillan).

Minuchin, S. and Fishman, H. C. (1981) *Family Therapy Techniques* (Cambridge, MA: Harvard University Press).

Moncrieff, J. (1999) 'An investigation into the precedents of modern drug treatments', *History of Psychiatry*, 10(40), 475–90.

Moncrieff, J. (2009) *The Myth of the Chemical Cure. A Critique of Psychiatric Drug Treatment* (Basingstoke: Palgrave Macmillan).

Moncrieff, J., Hopker, S. and Thomas, P. (2005) 'Psychiatry and the pharmaceutical industry: Who pays the piper? A perspective from the critical psychiatry network', *Psychiatric Bulletin*, 29, 84–5.

Mooney, G. (2012) 'Neoliberalism is bad for our health', *International Journal of Health Services*, 42(3), 383–401.

Morel, B-A. (1857) *Traité des dégénérescecs physique, intellectuelles et morales de l'espèce humaine* (Paris: Baillière). Cited by Shorter, 1997.

Morrison, T. (1993) *Playing in the Dark. Whiteness and the Literary Imagination* (London and Basingstoke: Pan Macmillan).

Murphy, G. (1938) *An Historical Introduction to Modern Psychology* (London: Routledge and Kegan Paul).

Murphy, H. B. M. and Raman, A. C. (1971) 'The chronicity of schizophrenia in indigenous tropical peoples', *British Journal of Psychiatry*, 118, 489–97.

Nakimuli-Mpungu, E., Alderman, S., Kinyada, E., Allden, K., Betancourt, T. S., Alderman, J. S., Pavia, Al., Okello, J., Nakku, J., Adaku, A. and Musisi, S. (2013) 'Implementation and scale-up of psycho-trauma centers in a post-conflict area: A case study of a private-public partnership in Northern Uganda', *PLOS Medicine*, 10(4), 1–8. Retrieved 20 April 2013 from: http://www.plosmedicine.org/

Narayan, D., Chambers, R., Shah, M. K. and Petesch, P. (2000) *Voices of the Poor; Crying Out for Change* (Oxford and New York: Oxford University Press).

Navarro, V. (1998) 'Neoliberalism, "Globalization," unemployment, inequalities, and the welfare state', *International Journal of Health Services*, 28(4), 607–82.

Navarro, V. (2007) 'Neoliberalism as a class ideology; Or the political causes of the growth of inequalities', *International Journal of Health Services*, 37(1), 47–62.

Navarro, V. (2009) 'What we mean by social determinants of health', *International Journal of Health*, 39(3), 423–41.

Ndegwa, D. and Olajide, (D. (eds) (2003) *Main Issues in Mental Health and Race*. Aldershot (Hants): Ashgate.

Neki, J. S. (1973) 'Psychiatry in South-East Asia', *British Journal of Psychiatry*, 123(3), 257–69.

Nelson, G. and Prilleltensky, I. (2005) *Community Psychology in Pursuit of Liberation and Well-being* (Basingstoke: Palgrave Macmillan).

Ng, V. W. (1990) *Madness in Late Imperial China. From Illness to Deviance* (Norman, Oklahoma and London: University of Oklahoma Press).

Nichter, M. (1980) 'The layperson's perception of medicine as perspective into the utilization of multiple therapy systems in the Indian context', *Social Science and Medicine*, 14B, 225–233.

Nichter, M. (1981) 'Idioms of distress: Alternatives in the expression of psychosocial distress: A case study from South India', *Culture, Medicine and Psychiatry*, 5(4), 379–408.

Nichter, M. (2010) 'Idioms of distress revisited', *Culture, Medicine and Psychiatry*, 34(2), 401–16.

NIMH (National Institute for Mental Health)/MHF (Mental Health Foundation) (2003) *Inspiring Hope: Recognizing the Importance of Spirituality in a Whole Person Approach to Mental Health* (Leeds: NIMHE).

Nobles, W. W. (1986) 'Ancient Egyptian thought and the renaissance of African (Black) psychology', in M. Karenga and J. H. Carruthers (eds) *Kemet and the African Worldview. Research, Rescue and Restoration* Part 3 (Los Angeles: University of Sankore Press) pp. 100–18.

O'Riordan (1998) 'Civic science and the sustainability transition', in D. Warburton (ed) *Community and Sustainable Development Participation in the Future* (London: Earthscan Publications) pp. 96–116.

Obeyesekere, G. (1977) 'The theory and practice of psychological medicine in the ayurvedic tradition', *Culture, Medicine and Psychiatry*, 1, 155–81.

Obeyesekere, G. (1985) 'Depression, Buddhism, and the work of culture in Sri Lanka', in A. Kleinman and B. Good (eds) *Culture and Depression* (Berkeley, CA: University of California Press) pp. 134–52.

Obeyesekere, G. (1990) *The Work of Culture. Symbolic Transformations in Psychoanalysis and Anthropology* (London and Chicago: University of Chicago Press).

Offer, D. and Sabshin, M. (1966) *Normality: Theoretical and Clinical Concepts of Mental Health* (New York: Basic Books).

Okasha, A. and Ashour, A. (1981) 'Psycho-demographic study of anxiety in Egypt: The PSE in its Arabic version', *British Journal of Psychiatry*, 139, 70–3.

Orley, J. and Wing, J. (1979) 'Psychiatric disorders in two African villages', *Archives of General Psychiatry*, 36, 513–20.

Owen, G. S., Szmukler, G., Richardson, G., David, A. S., Hayward, P., Rucker, J., Harding, D. and Hotopf, M. (2009) 'Mental capacity and psychiatric in-patients: Implications for the new mental health law in England and Wales', *British Journal of Psychiatry*, 195, 257–63.

Oxman, A. D., Lavis, J. N. and Fretheim, A. (2007) 'Use of evidence in WHO recommendations', *Lancet*, 369, 1883–9.

Parthasarathi, P. (2011) *Why Europe Grew Rich and Asia Did Not. Global Economic Divergence, 1600–1850* (Cambridge: Cambridge University Press).

Patel, V. and Prince, M. (2010) 'Global mental health. A new global health field comes of age', *Journal of the American Medical Association*, 303(19), 1976–77.

Patterson, D. K. 1981. *Health in Colonial Ghana: Disease, Medicine and Socio-Economic Change 1900–1955* (Waltham: Crossroads Press). Cited by Read, 2012.

Pearsall, J. and Trumble, B. (1995) *The Oxford English Reference Dictionary* (Oxford: Oxford University Press).

Pedersen, D., Kienzler, H. and Gamarra J. (2010) *Llaki* and *Ñakary*: Idioms of distress and suffering among the Highland Quechua in the Peruvian Andes', *Culture, Medicine and Psychiatry*, 34(2), 279–300.

Perera, R. (2011) 'How indigenous medical practitioners deal with mental illness', in S. Fernando and C. Weerackody (eds) *Aspects of Mental Health in Sri Lanka* (Colombo, Sri Lanka: People's Rural Development Association – PRDA) pp. 84–101.

Perera, R. and Hettiarachchi, L. (2011) 'Perceptions of mental illness in two tsunami affected communities in the South', in S. Fernando and C. Weerackody (eds) *Aspects of Mental Health in Sri Lanka* (Colombo, Sri Lanka: People's Rural Development Association – PRDA) pp. 35–57.

Petras, J. and Veltmeyer, H. (2001) *Globalization Unmasked. Imperialism in the 21st Century* (London: Zed Books).

Pick, D. (1989) *Faces of Degeneration. A European Disorder, c. 1848–c. 1918* (Cambridge: Cambridge University Press).

Pieterse, J. N. (1995) 'Globalization as hybriditization', in M. Featherstone, S. Lash and R. Robertson (eds) *Global Modernities* (London and New Delhi: Sage) pp. 45–68.

Pieterse, J. N. (2007) *Ethnicities and Global Multiculture. Pants for an Octopus* (Plymouth UK, New York and Toronto: Rowman and Littlefield).

Pieterse, J. N. (2009) *Globalisation and Culture. Global Mélange* (Plymouth UK, New York and Toronto: Rowman and Littlefield).

Pinel, P. (1806) *A Treatise on Insanity: In Which Are Contained the Principles of a New and More Practical Nosology of Maniacal Disorders That Has Yet Been Offered to the Public*. Reprinted 2010 by General Books Memphis Tennesse. Printed by Todd for Cadell and Davies 2010.

Pomeranz, K. (2001) *The Great Divergence: China, Europe and the Making of the Modern World Economy*, new edn. (Princeton: Princeton University Press).

Porter, B. (2012) *The Lion's Share. A History of British Imperialism 1850 to the Present*, 5th edn. (Harlow: Pearson Education).

Porter, R. (2002) *Madness. A Brief History* (Oxford and New York: Oxford University Press).

Prakash, G. (1990). 'Writing post-orientalist histories of the third world: Perspectives from Indian historiography', *Comparative Studies in Society and History*, 32(2), 383–408. doi:10.1017/S0010417500016534.

Prilleltensky, I., Nelson, G. and Peirson, L. (eds) (2001) *Promoting Family Wellness and Preventing Child Maltreatment: Fundamentals for Thinking and Action* (Toronto: University of Toronto Press).

Prince M., Patel V., Saxena S., Maj M., Maselko J., Phillips M. R., and Rahman, A. (2007) 'Health without mental health', *Lancet*, 370, 859–77.

Rack, P. (1982) *Race, Culture and Mental Disorder* (London and New York: Tavistock).

Raguram, R., Venkateswaram, A., Ramakrishna, J. and Weiss, M. (2002) 'Traditional community resources for mental health: A report of temple healing from India', *British Medical Journal*, 325, 38–40.

Ramon, S. and Williams, J. E. (eds) (2005) *Mental Health at the Crossroads. The Promise of the Psychosocial Approach* (Aldershot, Hants: Ashgate).

Read, U. (2012) *Between chains and vagrancy: Living with mental illness in Kintampo, Ghana*, Thesis presented for a research degree in Anthropology at University College, London.

Report of the Superintendent of Medical Services (1896) *The Lunatic Asylum, Jawatte* (Colombo, Sri Lanka: Government Printer, Ceylon).

Repper, J. and Perkins, R. (2003) *Social Inclusion and Recovery: A Model for Mental Health Practice* (London: Ballière Tindall).

Rinpoche, R. and Kunzang, J. (1973) *Tibetan Medicine* (London: Wellcome Institute of the History of Medicine).

Robertson, R. (1992) *Globalization Social Theory and Global Culture* (London and New Delhi: Sage).

Robertson, R. (1995) 'Glocalization: Time-space and homogeneity-heterogeneity', in M. Featherstone, S. Lash and R. Robertson (eds) *Global Modernities* (London and New Delhi: Sage) pp. 25–44.

Rodney, W. (1988) *How Europe Underdeveloped Africa* (London: Bogle L'Overture Publications).

Roger, P. (1994) 'Individuality in french enlightenment thought: Exaltation or denial?', in S. Bagge (ed) *Culture and History. The Individual in European Culture* (Cambridge MA: Scandinavian University Press) pp. 72–83.

Rosen, G. (1968) *Madness in Society* (New York: Harper and Row).

Rush, B. (1818) *Medical Inquiries and Observations upon the Disease of the Mind*, 2nd edn. (Philadephia: Richardson).

Ryle, G. (1990) *The Concept of Mind* (London: Penguin Books). First published by Hitchingson, New York, 1949.

Sachs, J. (2005) *The End of Poverty; How We Can Make it Happen in Our Lifetime* (Harmondsworth: Penguin).

Sachs, L. (1989) 'Misunderstanding as therapy: Doctors, patients and medicines in a rural clinic in Sri Lanka', *Culture, Medicine and Psychiatry*, 13, 335–49.

Safaya, R. (1976) *Indian Psychology* (New Delhi: Munshiram Manoharlal).

Said, E. W. (1994) *Culture and Imperialism* (London: Vintage).

Saraceno, B. (2004) 'Foreword', in World Health Organisation (ed) *Prevention of Mental Disorders. Effective Interventions and Policy Options*. A Report of the WHO Department of Mental Health and Substance Abuse in collaboration with the Prevention Research Centre of the Universities of Nijmergen and Maastricht (Geneva: WHO).

Sartorius, N., Gulbinat, W., Harrison, G., Laska, E., and Siegel, C. (1996) 'Long-term follow-up of schizophrenia in 16 countries', *Social Psychiatry and Psychiatric Epidemiology*, 31, 249–58.

Sartorius, N., Jablensky, A., Korten, A., Ernberg, G., Anker, M., Cooper, J. E. and Day, R. (1986) 'Early manifestations and first-contact incidence of schizophrenia in different cultures: A preliminary report on the initial evaluation phase of the WHO collaborative study on determinants of outcome of severe mental disorders', *Psychological Medicine*, 6, 909–28.

Sax, W. S. (2009) *God of Justice. Ritual Healing and Social Justice in the Central Himalayas* (Oxford: Oxford University Press).

Saxena, S., Jane-Llopis, E., and Hosman, C. (2006) 'Prevention of mental and behavioural disorders: Implications for policy and practice', *World Psychiatry*, 5(1), 5–14.

Sayce, L. and Perkins, R. (2000) 'Recovery: Beyond mere survival', Letter to editor, *Psychiatric Bulletin*, 24, 74.

Scheff, T. J. (1966) *Being Mentally Ill: A Sociological Theory* (Chicago: Aldine).

Scott, J. and Beck, A. A. (2008) 'Cognitive behavioral therapy', in R. M. Murray, K. S. Kendler, P. McGuffin, S. Wessely and D. J. Castle (eds) *Essential Psychiatry*, 4th edn. (Cambridge: Cambridge University Press).

Scott, R. D. (1960) 'A family-orientated psychiatric service to the London borough of Barnet', *Health Trends*, 12, 65–8.

Scull, A. (1977) *Decarceration. Community Treatment and the Deviant. A Radical View* (Eaglewood Cliffs NJ: Prentice Hall).

Scull, A. (1984) *Decarceration. Community Treatment and the Deviant. A Radical View*, 2nd edn. (Cambridge: Polity Press).

Scull, A. (2011) *Madness. A Very Short Introduction* (Oxford: Oxford University Press).

Self, W. (2013) 'Psychiatrists: The drug pushers', *The Guardian Review*, 3 August, pp. 2–3. Retrieved 3 August 2013 from: http://www.theguardian.com/society/2013/aug/03/will-self-psychiatrist-drug-medication

Sen, A. (1999) *Development as Freedom* (Oxford: Oxford University Press).

Sequeira, J. (1932) 'The brain of the East African native', *British Medical Journal*, 26 March, 581.

Shah, S. (2011) 'How private companies are transforming the global public health agenda', *Foreign Affairs*, 9 November 2011. Retrieved 23 March 2013 from: http://www.foreignaffairs.com/articles/136654/sonia-shah/how-private-companies-are-transforming-the-global-public-health.

Sharma, R. K. and Dash, V. B. (1983) *Agnivesa's Caraka Samhitā*, Text with English Translation and Critical Exposition, 2nd edn., vol. 1 (Varanasi, India: Choukhamba Sanskrit Series Office).

Sharma, R. K. and Dash, V. B. (1985) *Agnivesa's Caraka Samhitā*, Text with English Translation and Critical Exposition, 2nd edn., vol. 2 (Varanasi, India: Choukhamba Sanskrit Series Office).

Shoenberg, E. (ed.) (1972) *A Hospital Looks at Itself* (Plymouth: Cassirer).

Shorter, E. (1997) *A History of Psychiatry from the Era of the Asylum to the Age of Prozac* (New York: John Wiley).

SHSA (Special Hospitals Service Authority) (1993) *Report of the Committee of Inquiry into the Death in Broadmoor Hospital of Orville Blackwood and a Review of the Deaths of Two Other Afro-Caribbean Patients: 'Big, Black and Dangerous?'* (Chairman Professor H. Prins) (London: SHSA).

Shukla, A., Philip, A., Zachariah, A.... and Shatrugna, V. (2012a) 'Critical perspectives on the NIMH initiative 'Grand Challenges to Global Mental Health'', *Indian Journal of Medical Ethics*, 9(4), 292–3.

Shukla, A., Philip, A., Zachariah, A.... and Shatrugna, V. (2012b) 'Grand challenges to global mental health', *e-SocialSciences Current Affairs*, October 2012.

Shukla, A., Philip, A., Zachariah, A.Phadke, A....and others (2012c) 'Grand challenges for global mental health', *Economic and Political Weekly*, XLVIII (42), 4–5.

Simon, R. J., Fleiss, J. L., Gurland, B. J., Stiller, P. R. and Sharpe, L. (1973) 'Depression and schizophrenia in hospitalised black and white mental patients', *Archives of General Psychiatry*, 28, 509–12.

Sivayokan, S. (2011) 'Meanings beyond words: Expressions of distress in three communities in the North', in S. Fernando and C. Weerackody (eds) *Aspects of Mental Health in Sri Lanka* (Colombo, Sri Lanka: People's Rural Development Association – PRDA) pp. 58–83.

Smith, G. (2008) *A Short History of Secularism* (London and New York: Cambridge University Press).

Somasundaram, D. (2007) 'Collective trauma in Northern Sri Lanka: A qualitative psychosocial-ecological study', *International Journal of Mental Health Systems*, 1, 5–31.

Somasundaram, D. and Sivayokan, S. (2013) 'Rebuilding community resilience in a post-was context: Developing insight and recommendations – a qualitative study in Northern Sri Lanka', *International Journal of Mental Health Systems*, 7(3), 1–24.

Stanley, J. (2009) 'African and Caribbean mental health services in Manchester', in S. Fernando and F. Keating (eds) *Mental Health in a Multi-Ethnic Society. A Multidisciplinary Handbook,* 2nd edn. (London and New York: Routledge) pp. 204–216.

Steger, M. B. and Roy, R. K. (2010) *Neoliberalism. A Very Short Introduction* (Oxford and New York: Oxford University Press).

Summerfield, D. (2012) 'Afterword: Against "global mental health" ', *Transcultural Psychiatry*, 49(3), 1–12.

Swartz, L., Ben-Arie, O. and Teggin, A.F. (1985) 'Subcultural delusions and hallucinations. Comments on the Present State Examination in a multi-cultural context', *British Journal of Psychiatry*, 146, 391–94

Szasz, T. S. (1962) *The Myth of Mental Illness* (London: Secker and Warburg).

Tew, J. (2002) *Social Perspectives in Mental Health; Developing Social Models to Understand and Work with Mental Distress* (London: Jessica Kingsley).

Thomas, P. (2013) 'Soteria: Contexts, practice and philosophy', in S. Coles, S. Keenan and B. Diamond (eds) *Madness Contested Power and Practice* (Ross-on-Wye, Herefordshire: PCCS Books) pp. 141–57.

Thomas, A. and Sillen, S. (1972) *Racism and Psychiatry* (New York: Brunner/Mazel).

Thomas, P. (1997) *The Dialectics of Schizophrenia* (London and New York: Free Association Books).

Thomas, P., Bracken, P. and Timimi, S. (2012) 'The anomalies of evidence-based medicine in psychiatry: Time to rethink the basis of mental health practice', *Mental Health Review Journal*, 17(3), 152–62.

Thornicroft, G. and Tansella, M. (2004) 'Components of a modern mental health service: A pragmatic balance of community and hospital care', *British Journal of Psychiatry*, 185, 283–90.

Tischler, G. L. (1987) *Diagnosis and Classification in Psychiatry. A Critical Appraisal of DSM-III* (Cambridge: Cambridge University Press).

Tomlinson, B. R. (2003) 'What was the Third World?', *Journal of Contemporary History*, 38(2), 307–21.

Triandis, H. C. (1995) *Individualism and Collectivism* (Boulder and Oxford: Westview Press).

Tribe, R. (2007) 'Health pluralism: A more appropriate alternative to Western models of therapy in the context of the civil conflict and natural disaster in Sri Lanka?', *Journal of Refugee Studies*, 20(1), 21–36.

Trivedi, P. (2009) 'Black service' user involvement' – rhetoric or reality?', in S. Fernando and F. Keating (eds) *Mental Health in a Multi-Ethnic Society. A Multidisciplinary Handbook*, 2nd edn. (London and New York: Routledge) pp. 136–46.

Tuke, D. H. (1858) 'Does civilization favour the generation of mental disease?', *Journal of Mental Science*, 4, 94–110.

Tuke, D. H. (1890) 'French retrospect', *Journal of Mental Science*, 36(152), 117–122.

Tuke, S. (1813) *A Description of the Retreat, An Institution Near York, for Insane Persons of the Society of Friends* (York: W. Alexander).

United Nations (1948) *Universal Declaration of Human Rights*. General Assembly Resolution 217A (III), UN Doc. A/810 at 71 (New York: United Nations). Retrieved 12 June 2013 from: http://www1.umn.edu/humanrts/instree/b1udhr.htm.

Uragoda, C. G. (1987) *A History of Medicine in Sri Lanka – from the Earliest Times to 1948* (Colombo, Sri Lanka: Sri Lanka Medical Association).

Valiathan, M. S. (2003) *The Legacy of Caraka* (Hyderabad: Orient Longman).

Vige, M. (ed.) (2008) *Goodbye TCPS*, Special edition of Diverse Minds (London: Mind).

Vint, F. W. (1934) 'The brain of the Kenya native', *Journal of Anatomy*, 68, 216–23.

Vogt, B. (1999) *Skill and Trust: The Tovil Healing Ritual of Sri Lanka as Culture-Specific Psychotherapy*, Sri Lanka studies 6, trans. M. H. Kohn (Amsterdam: VU University Press).

Walvin, J. (1992) *Back Ivory. A History of British Slavery* (London: Fontana Press).

Warburton, D. (1998) 'A passionate dialogue: Community and sustainable development', in D. Warburton (ed) *Community and Sustainable Development Participation in the Future* (London: Earthscan Publications) pp. 1–39.

Warner, R. (1985) *Recovery from Schizophrenia* (New York, NY: Routledge and Kegan Paul).

Watters, E. (2011) *Crazy Like Us; The Globalization of the Western Mind* (London: Constable and Robinson).

Waxler, N. (1984) 'Behavioural convergence and institutional separation: An analysis of plural medicine in Sri Lanka', *Culture, Medicine and Psychiatry*, 8, 187–205.

Waxler-Morrison, N. E. (1988) 'Plural medicine in Sri Lanka: Do ayurvedic and western medical practices differ?', *Social Science and Medicine*, 27(5), 531–44.

Weaver, C. and Leiteritz (2005) ' "Our poverty is a world full of dreams": Reforming the World Bank', *Global Governance*, 11, 369–388.

Weber, M. M. and Engstrom, E. J. (1997) 'Kraepelin's "diagnostic cards": The confluence of clinical research and preconceived categories', *History of Psychiatry*, 8, 375–85.

Weerackody, C. and Fernando, S. (2008) 'Field Report. Perceptions of social stratification and well-being in refugee communities in North-Western Sri Lanka', *International Journal of Migration, Health and Social Care*, 4(2), 47–56.

Weerackody, C. and Fernando, S. (2011) *Reflections on Mental Health and Wellbeing Learning from Communities Affected by Conflict, Dislocation and Natural Disaster* (Colombo, Sri Lanka: People's Rural Development Association – PRDA).

Weiner, D. B. (1992) 'Philippe Pinel's "Memoir on Madness" of 11 December 1794: A fundamental text of modern psychiatry', *American Journal of Psychiatry*, 149(6), 725–732.

WFMH (World Federation for Mental Health) (2012) *Depression. A Global Crisis* (Occoquan, USA: WFMH).

Whitaker, R. (2002) *Mad in America* Perseus (Cambridge, MA: Publishing).

Whitaker, R. (2010) *Anatomy of an Epidemic. Magic Bullets, Psychiatric Drugs, and the Astonishing Rise of Mental Illness in America* (New York: Broadway paperbacks).

White, G. M. (1982) 'Ethnographic study of cultural knowledge of "Mental Disorder" ', in A. J. Marsella and G. M. White (eds) *Cultural Concepts of Mental Health and Therapy* (Dordrecht: Reidel) pp. 69–95.

WHO (World Health Organization) (1948) *The ICD-6 Classification of Mental and Behavioural Disorders* (Geneva: WHO).

WHO (World Health Organization) (1973) *Report of the International Pilot Study of Schizophrenia*, vol. 1 (Geneva: WHO).

WHO (World Health Organization) (1975) *Schizophrenia: A Multinational Study. A Summary of the Initial Evaluation Phase of the International Pilot Study of Schizophrenia* (Geneva: WHO).

WHO (World Health Organization) (1978) *Declaration of Alma-Ata*. International Conference on Primary health Care, Alma-Ata, USSR, 6–12 September 1978. Retrieved 20 April 2013 from: http://www.who.int/publications/almaata_declaration_en.pdf

WHO (World Health Organization) (1979) *Schizophrenia: An International Follow-up Study* (London: Wiley).

WHO (World Health Organization) (1986) *A Report on the Collaborative Study in Determinants of Outcome of Severe Mental Disorders.* Unpublished manuscript cited by Katz *et al.* 1988.

WHO (World Health Organization) (1988) *From Alma-Ata to the Year 2000 Reflections at the Midpoint* (Geneva: WHO_. Retrieved 12 June 2013 from: http://www.who.int/publications/almaata_declaration_en.pdf

WHO (World Health Organization) (1992) *ICD-10 Classification of Mental and Behavioural Disorders*: Clinical Descriptions and Diagnostic Guidelines (Geneva: WHO).

WHO (World Health Organization) (2001) *World Health Report 2001—Mental Health: New Understanding, New Hope* (Geneva: WHO). Retrieved 07 March 2013 from: http://www.who.int/whr/2001/en/

WHO (World Health Organization) (2002) *Nations for Mental Health. Final Report* (Geneva: WHO) Retrieved 10 July 2013 from: http://www.who.int/mental_health/media/en/400.pdf

WHO (World Health Organization) (2004) *Prevention of Mental Disorders. Effective Interventions and Policy Options,* A Report of the World Health Organization, Department of Mental Health and Substance Abuse in collaboration with the Prevention Research Centre of the Universities of Nijmergen and Maastricht (Geneva: WHO). Retrieved 12 June 2013 from: http://www.who.int/mental_health/evidence/en/prevention_of_mental_disorders_sr.pdf

WHO (World Health Organization) (2008a) *mhGAP: Mental Health Gap Action Programme: Scaling up Care for Mental, Neurological and Substance use Disorders,* Geneva: WHO. Retrieved 09 April 2013 from: http://www.who.int/mental_health/evidence/mhGAP/en/index.html.

WHO (World Health Organization) (2008b) 'Mental health' *WHO.* Retrieved 20 April 2013 from: http://www.who.int/topics/mental_health/

WHO (World Health Organization) (2010) 'Mental disorders' *WHO* Retrieved 15 July 2013 from: http://www.who.int/topics/mental_disorders/en/

WHO (World Health Organization) (2011a) *All for Equity. World Conference on Social Determinants of Health.* Meeting Report Rio de Janeiro, Brazil 19–20 October 2011 (Geneva: WHO). Retrieved 20 April 2013 from: http://www.who.int/sdhconference/resources/Conference_Report.pdf..

WHO (World Health Organization) (2011b) *Consultation on Implementing Action on Social Determinants of Health to Reduce Health Inequities: The Contribution of Collaborative Work between Sectors.* Meeting Report (Geneva: WHO). Retrieved 10 June 2013 from: http://www.who.int/whr/2001/en/whr01_en.pdf

WHO (World Health Organization) (2012) *Global Burden of Mental Disorders and the Need for a Comprehensive, Coordinated Response from Health and Social Sectors at the Country Level.* Report by The Secretariat to World Health Organisation sixty-fifth World health Assembly, Provisional agenda item 13.2 (Geneva: WHO).

WHO Regional Office for South-East Asia (2008). *Broad Regional Strategy for Non-communicable Diseases and Mental Health; Mental Health and Substance Abuse.* Retrieved 15 September 2008 from: http://www.searo.who.int (No longer available on a website).

WHO/UNICEF (1978) *Primary Health Care: The Alma Ata Conference* (Geneva: WHO).

Wilkinson, R. and Picket, K. (2010) *The Spirit Level* (London: Allen Lane).

Willetts, P. (2013) 'NGO: What's that?', *Quarterly Journal of the Royal Over-Seas League (ROSL),* March–May 2013, 6–7.

Wing, J. K. (1978) *Reasoning about Madness* (Oxford: Oxford University Press).

Wing, J. K., Cooper, J. E. and Sartorius, N. (1974) *Measurement and Classification of Psychiatric Symptoms* (London: Cambridge University Press).

World Bank (2000) *Our Dream: A World Free of Poverty* (Washington DC: Oxford University Press and World Bank).

World Bank (2013) 'How we classify countries', *The World Bank.* Retrieved 23 April 2013 from: http://data.worldbank.org/about/country-classifications.

Wu, D, Y. H. (1984) 'Psychotherapy ad emotion in traditional Chinese medicine', in A. J. Marsella and G. M. White (ed) *Cultural Conceptions of Mental Health and Therapy* (Dordrecht: Kluwer) pp. 285–301.

Young, A. (1995) *The Harmony of Illusions. Inventing Post-Traumatic Stress Disorder* (Princeton NJ: Princeton University Press).

Zilborg, G. (1941) *A History of Medical Psychology* (New York: Norton).

Author Index

Subject Index

Note: locators in **bold** refer to tables in the text

Printed and bound by CPI Group (UK) Ltd, Croydon, CR0 4YY